THE

Natural Healing & Nutrition

ANNUAL

1993

THE
Natural Healing & Nutrition
ANNUAL
1993

Edited by Mark Bricklin, Editor,
PREVENTION Magazine,
& Matthew Hoffman,
PREVENTION Magazine Health Books

Rodale Press, Emmaus, Pennsylvania

Our Mission

We publish books that empower people's lives.

RODALE BOOKS

Contributors to
The Natural Healing and Nutrition Annual 1993

Writers: Pamela Boyer, Michael Castleman, Lisa
   Delaney, Stephanie Ebbert, Anne M. Fletcher, Greg
   Gutfeld, Alice Jurish, Steven Lally, Eileen Nechas,
   Connie Nesteruk, Cathy Perlmutter, Maggie
   Spilner, Sharon Stocker, Margo Trott, Susan Zarrow

Production Editor: Jane Sherman
Book and Cover Designer: Greg Imhoff
Layout Design: Ayers/Johanek Publication Design
Associate Research Chief, *Prevention* Magazine: Pam Boyer
Office Manager: Roberta Mulliner
Office Personnel: Julie Kehs, Mary Lou Stephen

Contents

■   ■

America's Favorite Home Remedies: The Best by Home Test

Nutrition and Health Updates

Contents

Eating for a Healthier Life

Medical Care Updates

The Power of Exercise

ix

Looking Good

Beating Disease

Emotional Fitness

Do It Naturally

Everyday Health Tips

The Good Life

SUPPLEMENTS AND COMMON SENSE

Some of the reports in this book give accounts of the professional use of nutritional supplements. While food supplements are in general quite safe, some can be harmful if taken in very large amounts. Be especially careful not to take more than these commonsense daily limits:

Vitamin A	2,000 IU
Vitamin B_6	50 mg
Vitamin D	400 IU
Selenium	100 mcg

NOTICE

The information and ideas in this book are meant to supplement the care and guidance of your physician, not to replace it. The editor cautions you not to attempt diagnosis or embark upon self-treatment of serious illness without competent professional assistance. An increasing number of physicians are ready to cooperate with clients who want to improve their diet and lifestyle; if you are under professional care or taking medication, we suggest discussing this possibility with your doctor.

Introduction

■   ■

For Good Health, You Need a Plan

Wouldn't it be wonderful if we could take the entire world of medical knowledge—the latest research, the newest findings, the best treatments—and squeeze it into one package? Not a magic pill, exactly, but a plan—a blueprint for beating disease and living a fuller, healthier life.

Here is the plan: *The Natural Healing and Nutrition Annual 1993.* You won't find magic bullets here. What you will find are hundreds of simple tips you can use every day.

You know that eating a low-fat, high-fiber diet is good for you. But did you also know it may reduce your risk for breast cancer? Researchers have found that eating carrots—and other vegetables high in vitamin A and beta-carotene—can help prevent cataracts. The same nutrients may put the brakes on some types of cancer. Even barley flour may play a role in lowering cholesterol and preventing heart disease.

You can't have a good-health plan without exercise. That's why we've included an entire section on walking, weight training, even dancing! (We'll give you some tips for beating perspiration, too.)

As a bonus, we've included a special report on *Prevention* Magazine's Home-Remedy Survey. Thousands of people were asked about their favorite home remedies—everything from ginger for motion sickness to hot baths for muscle aches. Learn which worked best—and which fell flat!

For your dining pleasure, we've included the winning recipes from *Prevention*'s Low-Fat Cook-Off. Now you can enjoy delicious, easy-to-prepare meals every day.

The truth is, there's nothing difficult about achieving—and maintaining—good health. All you need is a plan. Here it is. Enjoy!

The Editors
Prevention Magazine

America's Favorite Home Remedies

THE BEST BY HOME TEST

Healing
with Food

Nature's all-purpose medicine chest is brimming with relief.

People rely heavily on dietary therapies for minor upsets as well as chronic conditions. In this survey, over 3,300 respondents said they tried bran or fiber cereal to relieve constipation, for example, and roughly the same number said they tried a low-fat diet to lose weight.

And that's a good sign, says Jay Kenney, R.D., Ph.D., a nutrition research specialist at the Pritikin Longevity Center in Santa Monica, California. "The focus really should be on using foods or diet instead of drugs when they work equally well—or even better."

This overwhelming interest in dietary alternatives comes as no surprise to experts. "It's human nature," says Ara H. DerMarderosian, Ph.D., professor of pharmacognosy and medicinal chemistry at the Philadelphia College of Pharmacy and Science. "People prefer to do something simple, easy and inexpensive."

Food is comforting, familiar territory, and changing your diet to include more of one thing or less of another really involves little or no extra work—you've got to eat something, after all.

The idea appeals to doctors and scientists as well. This approach has become one of the hottest areas of medical research. In fact, the National Cancer Institute is taking this approach one step further. Instead of recommending just cutting out harmful elements of the diet or adding helpful ones, its Designer Foods Research Project is working to identify any powerful anticancer substances in certain foods and then find ways to concentrate them and test them against the disease.

We won't see the results of that project for many years. But clearly, medicine has decided that food is more than just sustenance. Doctors know that by tailoring your diet to combat certain problems—high blood pressure or high cholesterol—you can bring about enormous changes in your health. And this method doesn't carry the risk of side effects that drug therapies can.

In this survey, food remedies were rated "good," "fair" or "poor." The survey results and anecdotes should not be construed as scientific evidence—the most reliable guide for effectiveness. They're merely a report of how well people said the food remedies worked for them. However, many of the food remedies are backed by solid scientific research—controlled studies in which the remedy faced off against a placebo (an inactive look-alike). Here's what people had to say about how well food remedies worked for them.

Bran for Constipation

People gave bran and high-fiber cereal top honors for relieving irregularity. Eighty-six percent of those who tried it reported "good" results—the highest of any food remedy in the survey. Another 12 percent said they got "fair" results.

"I am 63 years old and never have to take laxatives," said a woman from Waverly, Ohio. "High-fiber cereal—and walking—keeps things 'going.'" Another respondent said, "We use miller's bran to relieve constipation (my husband and I). And I have relief from hemorrhoids when I use bran. If I miss my bran, hemorrhoids bother me again."

These successes come as no surprise, for the benefits of whole-grain foods have been known since ancient times—and have been confirmed by science. If you're planning to jump on the bran wagon, stick to coarse bran rather than bran that's ground to a fine powder, says Dr. Kenney. "Finely ground bran has much less of an effect on constipation."

And here are some general pointers for beefing up your fiber intake: Boost your intake gradually to give your system a chance to adjust. "Bran or high fiber works better if you drink the daily requirement of water," added a Philadelphia correspondent. Drinking at least eight eight-ounce glasses a day is important because fiber soaks up fluids.

A Low-Fat Diet to Lose Weight

Some food remedies require eating not more of a good thing but less of a bad one. "In fact, most of the health gains people can get from improving nutrition are by reducing or eliminating substances that have negative effects," says Dr. Kenney. A case in point: fat.

Eighty-two percent of those who tried a low-fat diet to reduce weight reported good success—second only to bran among the food remedies.

"I think this percentage is appropriate," says George Blackburn, M.D., Ph.D., associate professor at Harvard Medical School and chief of the Nutrition/Metabolism Laboratory at New England Deaconess Hospital, Boston. "The reason it isn't 100 percent reflects the difficulty that many people have in ferreting out the fat in their diet. Half of it is hidden—in restaurant meals and processed foods, for example. If we were perfect at following it, a truly low-fat diet (less than 25 percent of calories from fat) would be 100 percent effective for weight loss."

Many large research studies have shown that low-fat diets cause pounds to drop off. Some showed that it's not just the reduction in calories that causes weight loss—it's also the reduction in fat.

In a study of over 300 normal-weight women at centers in Seattle, Houston and Cincinnati, women who ate a very-low-fat diet (20 percent of calories from fat) lost weight even though they were allowed to eat whatever else they wanted.

"Over two years on a low-fat, moderate-protein, high-carbohydrate diet with moderate, regular exercise has allowed me to lose 92 pounds," said a woman from Durham, North Carolina. "It works!"

"A low-fat diet for weight loss is excellent," said a Columbus, Ohio, correspondent. "My brother has lost 100-plus pounds in a year using this approach."

A Low-Fat Diet to Lower Cholesterol

Fifty-five percent of the respondents tried this dietary maneuver, with 82 percent reporting "good" results.

"A low-fat diet helped lower my cholesterol by over 100 points," said a man from Library, Pennsylvania.

"I'm no pill taker," said another correspondent. "I control my high cholesterol with diet and exercise."

"I'm a little surprised that only 82 percent reported good results," says Dr. Kenney, "because here at the Pritikin Center, more than 95 percent of the people have success on a low-fat diet. The difference can probably be explained by the degree of diet changes. We keep total fat to around 10 percent of calories. We also keep saturated fat, in particular, and cholesterol extremely low." At home, people may not be lowering their fat intake enough. And they may not be cutting dietary cholesterol enough.

Probably hundreds of studies have shown that a low-fat diet reduces cholesterol. To embark on a low-fat diet, concentrate on fruits, vegetables, whole grains and other complex carbohydrates.

A Low-Caffeine Diet to Reduce Anxiety

"Cutting out caffeine completely from my diet really helped reduce stress and anxiety," said one survey respondent.

"A no-caffeine diet eliminated hand tremors and anxiety," said another.

That was the prevailing attitude, as 79 percent of those who tried it agreed. Forty-seven percent of the respondents gave this a try.

"This makes all the sense in the world," says Redford Williams, M.D., professor of psychiatry and director of the Behavioral Medicine Research Center at Duke University Medical Center. "It's not uncommon to advise people who seem 'charged up' to lay off caffeine, simply because it's a stimulant. Often, doing that helps reduce anxiety."

In fact, caffeine has been found to cause panic attacks in some people who have panic disorder. "Other research shows that drinking the amount of caffeine in a single cup of coffee enhances the body's physical responses to

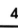

stress, such as raising blood pressure even higher," says Dr. Williams. "This suggests that caffeine is probably doing something to increase the activity in our sympathetic nervous system, which maintains our fight-or-flight response. So cutting out caffeine should be helpful in reducing our responses to stress."

If you're trying to cut back or eliminate caffeine, try substituting a caffeine-free product for your coffee or cola, says Dr. Williams, so you won't miss the taste. You may also want to reduce caffeine gradually because there can be withdrawal symptoms including headaches and nausea.

A Low-Sodium Diet to Reduce Blood Pressure

"My blood pressure stays normal with the no-salt diet," said a correspondent from Falmouth, Massachusetts.

Seventy-seven percent of the survey respondents who tried this agreed—reporting "good" results.

"It surprises me that their success rate is so high," says Dr. Kenney. "Generally, only about 50 percent of people with high blood pressure who reduce dietary salt alone see their blood pressure go down, unless the sodium reduction is extreme.

"The important thing to note, though, is that the vast majority of people who develop high blood pressure do so to a large extent because there is salt in the diet. Populations that add no salt to their food throughout their entire lifetime do not get hypertension, and blood pressure does not rise with age, whereas every population that adds salt to their food does see blood pressure rise with age.

"And we know from animal studies," says Dr. Kenney, "that when you feed animals a high-salt diet and create hypertension in them, and then put the animals on a low-salt diet, the hypertension does not always reverse. So it seems that excess salt can cause permanent damage. However, those who go on a low-salt diet before they develop hypertension stand an excellent chance of avoiding it."

Most experts recommend a sodium ceiling of 1,500 to 2,000 milligrams per day in a low-sodium diet, roughly the amount in one teaspoon of salt.

Fiber to Reduce Blood Cholesterol

Both oat bran and psyllium have proven to be potent cholesterol reducers. Seventy percent of those who tried eating oat bran or oatmeal to reduce cholesterol said they got good results (53 percent of the respondents tried this). Sixty-seven percent of those who tried psyllium said their cholesterol level dropped (but only 17 percent gave this a shot).

But those who said they tried other fiber-rich foods to lower cholesterol met with the greatest success—75 percent said that when their intake went up, their cholesterol came down. (Forty-one percent tried this.)

"I'm not surprised that the people who tried to increase fiber-rich foods in their diet were more successful," says Dr. Kenney, "because they were probably substituting those foods, such as fruits, vegetables and beans, for foods high in saturated fat and cholesterol, such as meat. Those people would be getting a double benefit—more fiber and less fat and cholesterol. The people who used oat bran or psyllium, though, may have just been adding them to a diet that was high in fat and cholesterol."

"By following a low-fat, high-fiber diet, I have lost 20 pounds. And I lowered my cholesterol from 240 to 183," said one respondent. Added two others, "For cholesterol, we've combined the use of garlic, high-fiber foods, bran, exercise and a low-fat diet, and we credit cholesterol reduction to the combination."

Yogurt for Digestive Upsets and Cold Sores

Cool, creamy, refreshing—yogurt has a lot to recommend it. But people aren't eating it solely because it's pleasing to the palate. They consider it serious medicine and are enlisting this white knight of the dairy world in the fight against digestive upsets.

In the survey, 73 percent reported "good" relief from yogurt. The active ingredients in yogurt, acidophilus pills and acidophilus milk are "friendly" bacteria. And there's actually some scientific evidence that they can fend off diarrhea caused by antibiotics.

Normally, the good bacteria in your intestines outnumber the bad by about 99 to 1. But when you take antibiotics, the ratio shifts in favor of the bad bugs, with diarrhea being the result. When you eat yogurt or take acidophilus, which are teeming with "friendlies," you help shift the balance back.

One small study in France compared the effects of yogurt with live cultures of good bacteria with yogurt that had been heated to kill all the bacteria. Volunteers who were taking an antibiotic didn't know which yogurt they were getting. Nine out of ten volunteers who ate yogurt with live cultures suffered no diarrhea. But eight of ten volunteers who got heated yogurt did develop diarrhea. In addition, stool samples showed much fewer of the offending bacteria in those eating yogurt with live cultures.

Experts do caution, though, that people with serious intestinal woes like diverticulitis, colitis and chronic diarrhea should not substitute a home remedy for a physician's medical care.

Twenty percent of the survey respondents gave yogurt or acidophilus pills a chance to conquer cold sores, with 69 percent of them reporting good results.

The scientific research on yogurt, acidophilus and cold sores is very sketchy, however, and dates all the way back to the 1950s. Regardless, many people said yogurt and acidophilus helped them.

"I cannot tell you what a relief it was to find something to work on fever blisters," said a woman from Dallas. "I had suffered with them for years. Acidophilus works like a charm. If used at the first tingle, sometimes it completely wards them off."

Some people found success treating canker sores with this remedy as well. Said a man from Baton Rouge,

Louisiana, "I was plagued for many years by canker sores in the mouth, with as many as ten at a time. In just two days after taking acidophilus capsules, my mouth cleared up. I don't take capsules as a daily supplement, but only if the sores come back, about every four to six months."

Chicken Soup
for Congestion or Colds

Sixty-eight percent of the 5,000 survey respondents said they tried to liquidate a cold with this culinary cure. Seventy percent said it helped.

One small study showed that a cup of hot chicken soup got nasal mucus flowing better than a cup of cold water. Hot water also outperformed cold water, but as you might expect, it didn't do quite as well as chicken soup. Because drinking either through a straw was not as effective as sipping it from a cup, the researchers felt that the effect might be due, at least in part, to nasal inhalation of water vapor.

A Fremont, California, correspondent said, "The steam of chicken soup is its magic." While science hasn't provided any evidence that chicken soup can help cure a cold, it can't hurt. "At the very least, it helps replace fluids lost through fever and nose blowing during a cold," says Varro Tyler, Ph.D., professor of pharmacognosy at Purdue University.

The extra fluid also helps dilute the mucus in your nose and upper throat, which makes breathing easier. And it can be nutritious. "Just go easy on the salt or steer clear of high-sodium brands if you're going to continue this therapy for a long period of time," says Dr. Tyler.

Bananas for Diarrhea

We can only guess at the origin of this remedy, but it seems to have been around for some time. Said a woman from Palm Harbor, Florida, "Thirty-five years ago our doctor recommended bananas when our children had diarrhea."

While 32 percent of the survey respondents found the

banana cure appealing enough to give it a try, and a bunch of them (66 percent) reported success, there's really no evidence at all one way or the other.

"Bananas help replace some of the potassium lost during a bout of diarrhea," says Dr. DerMarderosian, "and their pectin (a soluble fiber) content should help the intestinal contents absorb fluid, making the stool less watery."

In any case, their use persists. "Many years ago our pediatrician recommended bananas, rice cereal and skim milk during diarrhea problems," said a woman from Spring Hill, Florida. "We have used it all these years. It works for adults, too."

A nurse from Horseheads, New York, said, "I use the BRAT diet—bananas, rice cereal, applesauce, toast—for diarrhea."

Fish or Fish Oil for Arthritis and Circulatory Problems

Researchers speculate that fish oil may interfere with the inflammation process in arthritis, possibly preventing flare-ups and slowing the progress of the disease.

In several suggestive but inconclusive studies, fish oil (rich in eicosapentaenoic acid, or EPA, an omega-3 fatty acid) outperformed olive oil (a "neutral" agent). People taking it had fewer arthritis symptoms related to inflammation—pain, morning stiffness and fatigue—than people taking olive oil did.

The speculation is that fish oil may help curb inflammation because it contains omega-3 fatty acids instead of omega-6's, which are abundant in other polyunsaturated fats. Although they are essential to health, omega-6 fatty acids can also be turned into inflammatory chemicals by your body. Omega-3's are turned into more benign products.

Twenty percent of those who wrote in said they tried this gift from the sea. Sixty-three percent of them said fish or fish oil did a "good" job of relieving arthritis.

A woman from Lookout Mountain, Tennessee, said, "After years of taking various medications for arthritis pains, I have been able to control them for the last five years by eating three cans of sardines a week."

Experts say that fish oil will never cure arthritis. At best, it can only block one of several inflammatory processes. "If there's any benefit, though, you can only get it by also eating less omega-6-containing polyunsaturates—that is, by being on a low-fat diet," says Dr. Blackburn. "And not just any fish will do. Only the deep-water fish, such as mackerel, tuna, salmon and bluefish, are high in EPA. A dietitian's guidance is advisable."

Fish oil's other possible benefits: Research shows it can lower triglycerides, a type of blood fat suspected of having a role in heart disease. Fish oil also makes blood platelets less sticky, which may decrease the chance of forming blood clots. But whether or not it can cause blood pressure to fall is yet to be established.

A Low-Fat Diet to Relieve Breast Pain

"A low-fat diet (20 to 30 grams per day) resulted in the easiest weight loss ever," said a woman from Alpine, California. "Also, I had been troubled with sore breasts for years. After starting the low-fat diet, the problem completely disappeared!"

Said a woman from Sherborn, Massachusetts, "I have cystic mastitis. Every annual checkup, I had to have a few cysts drained, plus, before my period, I experienced much breast pain. I have put myself on a very-low-fat diet for over a year. This year they found no cysts, and I am pain-free."

Twelve percent of those who took part in the survey tried this home remedy. Sixty-one percent of them said they got good results.

Actually, there is some evidence on this, but it's sketchy, and it involves only one kind of breast pain—cyclical mastopathy, which comes around the time of a woman's period. "There is no evidence, however, that any other type of breast pain may be helped by such a diet," says N. F. Boyd, M.D., head of the Division of Epidemiology and Statistics at the Ontario Cancer Institute in Toronto. A proper exam by your doctor can distinguish cyclical from noncyclical breast pain.

Herbal Healing 2

Remedies that worked for your grandparents will work for you, too.

Home remedies are practically a cottage industry. People say they use them on everything from everyday twists and scrapes to chronic conditions. In this survey, for example, more than 4,000 of the 5,000 people who responded said they tried aloe vera gel on a minor burn. Over 3,000 tried cranberry juice for a urinary infection.

"This suggests that there's tremendous interest in herbal remedies," says Ara H. DerMarderosian, Ph.D., professor of pharmacognosy and medicinal chemistry at the Philadelphia College of Pharmacy and Science. "But it also indicates a tremendous need for research on those remedies."

Indeed, there is an appalling lack of research on how well herbal remedies actually work—there has simply been little effort to find out.

While the survey did ascertain how well home remedies work for some people, these anecdotes are no substitute for scientific evidence. What's needed are controlled studies on herbal remedies—tests that pit the remedies against inactive look-alikes (placebos) in head-to-head contests. That would demonstrate how well they work (or don't work).

"If people report 80 percent success with a particular remedy, that's a pretty good tip-off that it's worth looking into, even if there is a considerable placebo effect," says Dr. DerMarderosian. "This survey may help lay the foundation for scientific research into the efficacy of herbal products in medical treatment."

Here's what people had to say about how well herbal remedies worked for them.

Aloe Vera

People gave the slippery gel squeezed from the aloe plant near-perfect marks in soothing and healing minor burns. Eighty-seven percent of those who tried it reported "good" results—the highest of any herbal remedy in the survey. Another 11 percent reported "fair" results.

"I'm not surprised at all," says Varro Tyler, Ph.D., professor of pharmacognosy at Purdue University. "Evidence seems to indicate that something in aloe gel inhibits the action of bradykinin, a peptide that produces pain in injuries like burns. It also inhibits the formation of thromboxane, a chemical detrimental to wound healing."

In one clinical trial, researchers from the University of Texas Medical Branch in Galveston applied a cream with aloe gel to patients with frostbite, which causes damage similar to that of a burn. Aloe healed them much more quickly than conventional treatment.

"I used aloe gel from the plant when I severely burned my leg on a hot motorcycle pipe," said a respondent from Staten Island, New York. "This was the only way to keep the pain away—it healed beautifully—and no scar, either."

And a correspondent from Spokane, Washington, said, "Aloe vera gel from the plant greatly relieved my husband's neck burns from radiation therapy. The time to healing was less than two days. Pain relief was instantaneous."

Many respondents said they keep an aloe plant in the kitchen. "Burns are common in my class," said a home-economics teacher from Bangor, Michigan. "Fresh aloe is the answer!"

People reported success using fresh aloe to relieve the pain of sunburn and bee stings, too. Many also said they can't bear to be parted from the plant—they even take an aloe leaf along on vacation.

While some people use aloe vera juice as a laxative, long-term internal use is not advisable. Aloe contains potent colon stimulants, and prolonged use can lead to lazy-bowel syndrome, when the bowel can no longer function normally on its own.

Cranberry Juice

From out of damp bogs come little red berries that many people believe thwart urinary infections. Seventy-eight percent of those who tried cranberry juice reported good results.

"I am prone to urinary tract infections, since many years ago I suffered a bout of cystitis that left a lot of scarring," said a woman from Murphysboro, Illinois. "Since then I've used cranberry juice, a small glass every morning, and I've never had a similar problem (with one exception—when I stopped drinking cranberry juice). An old family physician (who charged $5 a visit and made house calls) recommended it."

And a respondent from Bisbee, Arizona, expressed this popular sentiment: "I think cranberry juice may work better to prevent urinary infections than to cure them."

Yet a urologist from Shreveport, Louisiana, who participated in the survey says that in 30 years of practice "patients have never reported success" with cranberry juice.

Scientific work on cranberry juice has heated up lately, says Dr. Tyler. "They're finding that cranberry juice's action isn't due to its acid content, as folk wisdom has it, but to principles it contains that prevent infection-causing bacteria from adhering to the cells that line the bladder." Because they can't latch on, the theory goes, the bacteria flow out of the body with the urine. Evidence is still sketchy, but these findings may explain how cranberry juice might help prevent bladder infections. Some experts suggest, though, that the acidity of cranberry juice may further irritate a bladder that's already infected.

Cranberry juice is usually imbibed as a "cocktail" mixed with sugar (or sugar substitute) and water because it's highly acidic and too sour to drink straight. But one creative woman from Preston, Mississippi, relies on her own concoction: "Whole fresh cranberries and nonfat plain yogurt mixed in a blender with a little honey."

Garlic

Respondents agreed: This pungent herb is potent medicine. More than 37 percent of the 5,000 people who answered the survey had tried garlic for a cold or infection, with 70 percent reporting "good" results.

"Some studies from Italy and Greece showed that the

incidence of upper respiratory infections was fairly low in countries where they eat a lot of garlic," says Dr. DerMarderosian. And garlic does contain a compound that produces an antibiotic, allicin, when one of the cloves is cut or crushed.

"I swear that garlic taken at the first hint of a sore throat makes any cold go away," said a respondent from Cassiar, British Columbia. "I eat it roasted, boiled, stewed or fried, and all work. Fresh parsley helps to deodorize the garlic."

And a woman from Saco, Maine, added that although she believes it works as a preventive for her, "it didn't do much for me after I already had caught a cold."

More than 28 percent of the respondents had tried garlic for lowering cholesterol, and the same percentage had tried it for lowering blood pressure. In each case, roughly 69 percent of them reported favorable results.

"After one month on garlic, my blood pressure dropped from 164/92 to 130/78," said one respondent. Another reported that "within four weeks it changed from 155/90 to 135/80."

Animal research has shown that garlic can lower blood pressure, but no reliable studies with humans have surfaced. It's pretty well documented, however, that very high doses of garlic can lower cholesterol.

"Garlic and carrots are excellent for reducing cholesterol," said a woman from Maple Grove, Quebec. "These two vegetables did it for me."

But's there's one hitch. "The modern studies seem to indicate that to get real therapeutic value from garlic, you have to eat an awful lot of it, in excess of five cloves a day," says Dr. Tyler. "I don't think many people in this country eat that much."

Oil of Clove

This toothache remedy is strong medicine—so strong that in its pure form it can cause permanent nerve damage. That's why dentists don't use it on a tooth with a salvageable nerve. Over-the-counter preparations that contain clove oil (or its derivative, eugenol) in lesser concentrations are safe, though, if used according to package directions.

Thirty-seven percent of respondents said they tried clove oil for a toothache. Sixty-eight percent of them said they got relief.

"I'm surprised that that number wasn't higher," says Dr. Tyler. "Clove oil contains a proven anesthetic, eugenol. Perhaps those who didn't find relief didn't use the clove oil properly."

You have to get the clove oil on the nerve to deaden the pain, he says. So there has to be a cavity or crack through which the oil can penetrate to the nerve. Those who didn't get good results may have had an infection in the root or other condition for which clove oil is ineffective.

Even if clove oil works for you, it should be used only as a stopgap measure until you can get to a dentist. As a woman from Atlanta, Georgia, put it, "Oil of clove prolonged tooth problems because of my failure to visit a dentist." Another reported that it irritated her gums. Experts say that if your gums turn red, you've left the clove oil on too long.

Cherries

Fourteen percent of the respondents tried using cherries for gout, a form of arthritis that causes painful joint inflammation. Sixty-seven percent reported good results.

"It's surprising that people report such success with this remedy because there's not much documented evidence," says Dr. DerMarderosian. "There apparently have been no studies on this since the 1950s."

"Cherries for gout—it works for me," said a woman from Mildred, Pennsylvania. "I keep canned pie cherries on hand and try to eat them several times a week on cereal or dessert. When I don't eat them, I am in trouble."

Ginger

This traditional herbal remedy keeps delicate stomachs settled, said 67 percent of the respondents who tried it. And quite a few did try ginger to prevent nausea or

15
■

motion sickness: 22 percent of the 5,000 who wrote in.

There's some good evidence that ginger can prevent motion sickness. Researchers studied 36 rather courageous students who had motion sickness. The valiant volunteers swallowed either 940 milligrams of powdered ginger in capsules, 100 milligrams of Dramamine (a standard over-the-counter anti–motion sickness pill) or capsules containing an inactive herb. Then they went for a ride, blindfolded, on a chair that tilted and revolved. The ginger group endured two minutes longer than the OTC group and four minutes longer than the inactive herb group before becoming queasy.

In a study from Denmark, 40 rookie sailors took one gram of ginger in unmarked capsules. Another 40 new naval cadets took blank look-alikes. The ginger group fared better in a four-hour jaunt on the high seas.

Another Danish study found that powdered ginger root effectively reduced nausea and vomiting during pregnancy (hyperemesis gravidarum) that was severe enough to warrant hospitalization.

And British researchers found that powdered ginger prevented nausea following major surgery just as well as the standard drug used for that purpose in a study of 60 women.

"Scientists don't know how it works," says Dr. Tyler. "But there is evidence ginger affects the stomach directly, rather than working through the central nervous system, as anti–motion sickness drugs do."

"Ginger worked fine during a rough storm on a cruise," reported a woman from Reading, Pennsylvania. And a woman from Houston, Texas, felt she couldn't rate ginger "good," "fair" or "poor," as the survey requested. "Where is your 'Excellent, works every time' column? I would rate ginger for nausea as excellent," she said.

But another respondent had a quite different experience: "Ginger tablets did virtually nothing against motion sickness compared with Dramamine."

For many years, ginger ale has been used as a remedy for a mildly upset stomach, but it really contains very little ginger. You can purchase powdered ginger capsules from your health-food store or raid your spice rack and dissolve ¼ teaspoon of ginger in hot water to make tea. Or munch on a small piece of crystallized ginger.

Peppermint

The benefits of this herb may be greater than just fresh breath. In animal studies, its main constituent, menthol, relaxed the muscular "trapdoor" between the esophagus and the stomach, allowing gas to escape. In other words, it promoted burping. Peppermint oil lowers the surface tension of gas bubbles, so uncomfortable gas is more easily released. And it calms agitated stomach muscles that are in the throes of indigestion.

About 56 percent of survey respondents tried peppermint for gas or stomach upset. Sixty-three percent of them reported good success.

"Peppermint oil works better than anything for my upset stomach," said a correspondent from Fort Worth, Texas.

But those prone to heartburn should beware. Peppermint can actually cause the problem by allowing stomach acid to escape into the esophagus. As a correspondent from Turnersville, New Jersey, attested, "Peppermint gives me heartburn!" Others may find it irritating to the stomach.

Comfrey

Fifty-five percent of respondents who said they tried comfrey topically reported that their skin problems cleared up after using the herb. Only 12 percent had tried it, though.

All that science can vouch for is that comfrey contains allantoin, a product that facilitates cell growth and development.

"For stitches and swelling after childbirth, a comfrey-leaf poultice was great," said a woman from Farmington, Michigan.

"When our son played soccer, poultices of crushed comfrey helped his bruises," said a mother from Circle Pines, Minnesota.

There is good evidence, however, that comfrey taken internally for several months can cause liver damage. "It should be safe to use topically, as long as you don't put it on open wounds through which comfrey might be absorbed," says Dr. Tyler.

Chamomile

"Of all the properties of chamomile tea, the sleep-inducing effect is probably the least proven," says Dr. Tyler. That may explain the sketchy results respondents reported. Forty-two percent tried drinking chamomile tea to induce sleep, but only 55 percent thought it helped them off to dreamland. Several claimed that it relaxes them and "soothes their nerves." But chamomile is better known for its antispasmodic (anticramp) and anti-inflammatory properties.

Several people did note they were allergic to chamomile. In fact, chamomile, like ragweed, is a member of the daisy family and should be avoided by anyone allergic to ragweed. If you develop symptoms of hives, hay fever or asthma after drinking chamomile tea, skip this remedy.

Jewelweed

Only 53 percent of the people who applied jewelweed to a poison ivy rash said that they got good relief from the mother of all itches. (Only 7 percent of the respondents had tried this remedy.)

"Even though its use persists, jewelweed doesn't really seem to be that effective for poison ivy," says Dr. DerMarderosian.

Jewelweed isn't available commercially. If you want to try this remedy, says Dr. Tyler, your best bet is to use sap fresh from the plant.

Uva-Ursi

Also known as bearberry, this traditional herbal remedy for urinary infections was once listed as an official drug in the national formulary, says Dr. Tyler. "It contains arbutin, a chemical that breaks down under alkaline conditions to hydroquinone, an antiseptic and diuretic. It's useful for modest infections, but it works only if the urine is kept alkaline. Fresh fruit and vitamin C tend to make the urine acid."

That may be why only 53 percent of the people who tried this herb for a urinary infection found that things cleared up well. Only 5 percent of those who wrote in actually tried this remedy. Another hint for using uva-ursi properly: It must be taken as a cold tea to avoid its irritating tannins, says Dr. DerMarderosian. Soak the leaves in room-temperature water for 20 to 30 minutes.

Feverfew

"After suffering from migraines for 35 years, I began taking feverfew at the onset (visual aura) of a migraine," said a woman from Roseville, Illinois. "It prevents the headache, nausea and all. I wish I'd known about feverfew 35 years ago!"

And a fellow from Casscoe, Arkansas, said, "Feverfew is the only migraine preventive that I've ever found to work."

Unfortunately, though, these two are in the minority. Of the 7 percent of survey respondents who pitted feverfew against these head pounders, only 39 percent got good results—the poorest showing of all the herbal remedies.

Thirty-four percent reported fair results and 27 percent, poor. "This is surprising, since recent research suggests that it may be useful in preventing migraines," says Dr. DerMarderosian.

In a 1988 study, researchers in Nottingham, England, gave 30 migraine sufferers one capsule of feverfew per day. Another 30 migraineurs took blank (placebo) capsules. After four months, the groups switched capsules for another four months. While the participants were taking feverfew, the number of headaches was reduced by 24 percent compared with when they were taking the placebo. And the migraines that did occur were less painful.

19
■

Why did people get such poor results? "I think the problem may be that they were using an inferior product," says Dr. Tyler. "A recent study in Britain showed that the commercial feverfew products there varied tremendously in the amount of parthenolide, the active ingredient they contain. And the United States does not have a standard that commercially available feverfew must meet."

The best bet, he says, is chewing a few fresh leaves every day. If fresh leaves are unavailable or irritate your mouth, switch to the freeze-dried herb in capsules or tablets (heat-drying destroys parthenolide). Feverfew is another member of the daisy family, so those with ragweed allergy should avoid it.

3 Healing with Vitamins and Minerals

Tough fighters on the health front.

It's a fact that vitamins and minerals can cure diseases caused by deficiencies of those nutrients. Deficiency diseases, though, are rare in this country. But there's good evidence that some nutrients can help in the fight against other ills. Niacin (a B vitamin), for example, can lower blood cholesterol levels. Calcium may help prevent the bone-thinning disease called osteoporosis. Folic acid (another B vitamin) can help prevent a certain kind of birth defect.

Are there other nutrient remedies out there like these that haven't been proven yet, remedies that could become mainstream medical treatments? Probably. The only way to tell for sure if a remedy really works is to test it scientifically. But that process can begin with each person. The responses in this survey don't prove that a given remedy is safe and effective, but they may strongly suggest that it deserves honest, scientific scrutiny.

Survey respondents pointed out that not all home remedies are helpful. Some are harmful, and people should determine the safety of any home remedy before trying it. (Don't guess.) Most important, no one should use a home remedy instead of getting medical care for a serious problem. Here's the lowdown on the remedies people said work best for them.

Vitamin C

For Colds ▸ Vitamin C dominates the list of vitamin and mineral remedies people said work best. More than 3,200 survey respondents—78 percent—said they have fewer colds when they take regular doses of vitamin C. Another 76 percent said vitamin C helps reduce cold and infection symptoms.

Ever since Nobel Prize winner Linus Pauling first advocated vitamin C as a weapon in the war on the common cold, more than 20 years ago, researchers have been busy trying to verify that claim. But so far, they've found little evidence that C prevents colds—in fact, there are more studies that say it doesn't. But there is evidence that it can keep the sniffles, coughing and sneezing to a minimum and that low levels of vitamin C in the body may be related to bronchitis and wheezing.

"Some studies do show some small preventive effect," says Jeffrey Blumberg, Ph.D., professor of nutrition and associate director of the United States Department of Agriculture (USDA) Human Nutrition Research Center at Tufts University. "But when you take all the studies together, it doesn't look very promising. The reduction in symptoms and duration of colds is pretty phenomenal in itself. If vitamin C doesn't actually prevent them, that doesn't make it any less wondrous."

For Bleeding Gums ▸ "I took vitamin C for my bleeding gums, and it worked," said a respondent from Library, Pennsylvania. That experience was reported by more than 77 percent of survey respondents who tried it.

Years ago, loose teeth and bleeding gums were the

telltale signs of scurvy (caused by severe vitamin C deficiency). That was when the disease was more common. Today it's more likely that your bleeding gums are a red flag of gum disease, caused by the buildup of plaque and bacteria at the edges of your gums and just underneath them. But low levels of vitamin C in the body can make the problem worse—lack of C weakens the tiny blood vessels in your gums, making them bleed more readily.

But you can't cure gum disease with C alone. "The number-one home remedy for bleeding gums is brushing and flossing," says Winston Morris, D.M.D., a specialist in endodontics and orthodontics and coauthor of *Balanced Nutrition Plan for Dental Patients*. "Even with optimal nutritional health, if you don't get the plaque and bacteria off your teeth and gums, you will have periodontal disease. But it has been shown that the severity of gum disease and the rate at which it progresses is definitely related to a lack of nutrients, like vitamin C."

Vitamin E

For Leg Cramps ▶ A whopping 73 percent of respondents reported good luck with vitamin E for leg cramps, especially the non-circulation-related leg cramps that strike only at night. "My dad was finally able to sleep free of leg cramps by taking vitamin E every day," said one correspondent from Hutchinson, Kansas.

Chances are, Pop had nocturnal leg cramps. They're surprise-attack muscle contractions, usually confined to the calves. They make it hard for their victims—mostly middle-aged and older adults, pregnant women and people with vascular disease—to get a good night's sleep. Why the cramps occur is still anybody's guess. Doctors don't commonly prescribe vitamin E for the disorder because so far there are only a few inconclusive studies to back up the success stories. But since research has called into question the effectiveness of quinine, the standard treatment for nocturnal leg cramps, there may be more attention paid to the alleged effects of vitamin E.

Calcium

For Muscle Cramps or Spasms ▶ More than 2,000 survey respondents said they've tried bone-building calcium for painful muscle pangs, and almost 74 percent report success.

"In the past year, I informed seven people about calcium for leg cramps—it works every time!" said a man from Spokane, Washington.

"There may be a good physiologic basis for that," says Bess Dawson Hughes, M.D., chief of the Calcium and Bone Metabolism Laboratory at the USDA Human Nutrition Research Center at Tufts University. "It is very well recognized that even slightly low potassium and low calcium levels cause muscle cramps."

If you're running low on calcium, your muscles become more easily "excited," and that can cause spontaneous cramping.

For Bone or Joint Pain ▶ More than 70 percent of respondents said calcium is also good for aching bones or joints. A woman from Ohio wrote, "I started taking calcium, and in five months, all my joint pains were gone, and I've had no pains since."

"Calcium cleared up my joint and bone problems 40 years ago," said a pleased South Carolinian.

But again, scientific evidence is sparse. "Calcium, in those who are deficient, slows down bone loss, particularly in women 55 and older," says Dr. Hughes. "But there's no pain involved with bone loss without fractures."

There is, though, a theoretical link between long-term calcium supplementation and relief of back pain. Bone loss, over time, may cause compression fractures of the spine. So calcium supplements, in the long run, may provide relief for an aching back caused by calcium deficiency.

For High Blood Pressure ▶ Almost 55 percent of respondents said their blood pressure levels dipped to healthier levels with the help of calcium.

That less-than-overwhelming response is consistent

23

with the scientific evidence, which is still not conclusive. One study of 58,000 women showed that consuming 800 milligrams of calcium per day—plus 300 milligrams of magnesium a day—reduced the chance of developing high blood pressure by one-third over four years. But other studies—sometimes showing calcium-induced blood pressure drops, other times showing no effect—continue to provide mixed signals.

"Calcium is particularly good, it seems, in affecting normal age-related increases in blood pressure. But there are a lot of causes of high blood pressure that calcium may not have anything to do with," Dr. Blumberg says.

If you've had good luck with calcium, it may be that you're salt-sensitive—which means that your blood pressure rises with salt intake. Salt-sensitive people retain water, and excess water in the blood vessels may turn up the pressure, the theory goes.

A number of studies have suggested that calcium acts as a natural diuretic, making your body release water. Another theory suggests that dietary calcium prevents the release of hormones that make the smooth muscle cells lining the blood vessels contract. That keeps the vessels relaxed and may keep blood pressure down.

People at high risk of developing hypertension because of low calcium intake—including pregnant women, blacks and those who overindulge in alcohol—may require more than the Recommended Dietary Allowance (RDA). But researchers have yet to determine the optimum levels of calcium intake for high-risk groups. And boosting your calcium intake through your diet or supplements is not a safe substitute for prescribed blood pressure medication. Before you stop taking any blood pressure medication, talk it over with your doctor.

For Premenstrual Syndrome ▶ About half of the respondents said they use calcium to quash the physical and emotional symptoms of premenstrual syndrome. "I always use calcium with magnesium and find it so helpful for cramps that I told my gynecologist—who then suggested it to his other patients," wrote a woman from Cedar Rapids, Iowa. Some pilot research has been done in this area, but it's inconclusive. A large study is under way, though, which may provide some definitive answers.

For women past menopause, some experts up the RDA from 800 milligrams to 1,200 milligrams because of calcium's demonstrated effectiveness against osteoporosis. Stick close to those levels unless you're under a doctor's care. Too much calcium may cause constipation, kidney stones or kidney dysfunction and may inhibit your body's absorption of iron, zinc and other essential minerals.

For Gum or Tooth Pain ▸ More than half of the 421 respondents who tried it said calcium also got rid of their gum or tooth pain. There's no established link between calcium and tooth or gum pain, but Dr. Morris has a theory. As you know, calcium deficiency makes your bones deteriorate—and that includes the bony support of the tooth. Add that to an abundance of bacteria-filled plaque, and you've got pain, swelling and discomfort.

"So it's possible that if you are calcium deficient and you supply calcium in your diet, that may slow up the progression of periodontal disease, and therefore, you feel better," Dr. Morris speculates.

Again, though—just like fighting gum disease with vitamin C—plaque control should be your priority. And any chronic tooth or gum pain should be checked out by a dentist.

Vitamin B$_6$

And/or Magnesium, for Kidney Stones ▸ "I've had kidney stones all my life," wrote a 46-year-old woman from Georgia. "But since I've been taking B$_6$, I have not had an infection or stone in four years." Almost 68 percent of those who tried it agree that B$_6$, either alone or combined with magnesium, protects people prone to stones.

Kidney stones are pea- to golf ball–size, brittle chunks of mineral salts that form in the kidneys or in the tubes that link the kidneys to the bladder. These pain-producing nuggets are usually made up of calcium oxalate or calcium phosphate, a combination of the two or a conglomeration of other minerals. The research on B$_6$ and magnesium—in combination or acting separately—

suggests that they're most effective when pitted against calcium stones caused by too much oxalate in the urine.

Studies as far back as the early 1960s have suggested B_6 as a stone-preventer. And a long-term study showed that 40 milligrams of B_6, per day, over five years, got rid of the calcium-oxalate crystals in the urine of the 100 research subjects.

But magnesium supplements should be taken only with a doctor's approval, and they should always be taken with meals because they bind to the oxalate in food and prevent its absorption, says Alan Wasserstein, M.D., director of the Stone Evaluation Center at the Hospital of the University of Pennsylvania in Philadelphia. The levels needed to combat kidney stones are much higher than the RDA of 350 milligrams for adult men and 280 milligrams for adult women. And high doses of B_6 can be toxic. So talk to your doctor before you begin supplementing with either nutrient. Neither B_6 nor magnesium breaks up stones that already exist—each is merely a preventive.

For Carpal Tunnel Syndrome ▶ Sixty-six percent of respondents who tried vitamin B_6 said that it relieved this wrist-wrenching disease, carpal tunnel syndrome (CTS).

CTS occurs when injury or overuse puts pressure on the median nerve that passes through a narrow opening in your wrist bones. That causes pain, numbness and tingling in the hand, which can become sharp bolts of pain that shoot up into the elbow, upper arm and shoulder. Splints can provide some relief, but many people end up having surgery. Some people with CTS actually lose the use of their hands entirely.

"Vitamin B_6 does play a role in the maintenance and health of nerves. Carpal tunnel syndrome is a particular nerve function that goes awry, so B_6 may be useful," Dr. Blumberg says. "But not all carpal tunnel syndrome cases respond to vitamin B_6."

If you think you have CTS, see a doctor before you begin vitamin therapy. The levels of vitamin B_6 used to treat CTS are well above the RDA of 2 milligrams for men and 1.8 milligrams for women. Large doses taken over a long term can cause nerve damage.

Zinc

For Body Odor ► More than 68 percent of survey respondents who used zinc topically said it's the winner when it's pitted (pun intended) against body odor. It ranked ninth on the list of top vitamin remedies.

"Zinc supplements have worked very well in removing my teenagers' awful foot odor," a grateful mom from Arizona wrote.

"There has been no scientific evidence to support this notion at all," says Norman Levine, M.D., professor and chief of dermatology at the University of Arizona Health Sciences Center.

It's true that zinc is contained in some antiperspirants, where it helps prevent perspiration by acting directly on the sweat glands. But experts say that, when taken in oral form, it probably doesn't work the same way. Further research may provide some answers to this question.

The RDA for adult men is 15 milligrams, and women should get 12 milligrams a day. Experts say you shouldn't go above 15 milligrams a day without supervision because too much zinc could affect your immune system or cause stomach irritation and vomiting.

For Poison Ivy or Skin Irritations ► More than 67 percent of those who tried zinc paste said that it soothes the stinging itch of poison ivy or other skin problems. "But there's no obvious medical reason why zinc-containing products would have an effect," Dr. Levine says. "It's harmless, though, and if it works, I don't have any objection to it." Zinc oxide is an ingredient in calamine lotion, which has drying capabilities. (Calamine is best applied like makeup, say the experts—so thinly that you can't see it.)

Vitamin D

For Bone and Joint Pain ► Sixty percent said that they successfully found solace from bone and joint pain with vitamin D. "I used to have pain in my ankles and feet when I woke up in the morning," said a correspondent from Allison Park, Pennsylvania. "I couldn't walk without shuffling—I was unable to bend or flex my ankles. I tried vitamin D and calcium, and have no more pain."

Well, vitamin D does work with calcium to build bone. It helps your body use the calcium you get through your diet. If you're too low on D, you could develop osteomalacia, a bone-loss disorder that can be painful.

Besides the vitamin D-to-calcium-to-bone-loss connection, vitamin D's been much ignored by researchers. "Nobody's really looked at this per se," says F. Michael Gloth, M.D., assistant professor of medicine with the Division of Geriatric Medicine and Gerontology at Johns Hopkins University. "Vitamin D is virtually all over our bodies, yet research has focused almost exclusively on bone."

Bone pain caused by vitamin D deficiency is pretty rare, though. The RDA for adults is only 200 international units a day—readily available in D-fortified dairy products and cereals. You can also get your daily dose of D during a 30-minute walk in the sun, because sun-exposed skin helps the body produce its own vitamin D.

But if the danger of skin cancer is keeping you under cover, or if an illness has rendered you homebound, you might have to be more careful about getting enough D, Dr. Gloth says. Without a doctor's supervision, don't take more than one 400–international unit capsule a day—the standard dosage available over the counter. Long-term megadoses could cause kidney disease (including kidney stones), stomach problems and, conceivably, muscle spasms and heart problems. Any unexplained bone or joint pain is good cause for a visit to your doctor, Dr. Gloth says. "Some causes of bone or joint pain can be extremely serious, and if you wait too long, it could be dangerous."

4   Holistic Healing

*Dozens of techniques for healing with
mind and body.*

"The wise, for cure, on exercise depend." The 17th-century English poet John Dryden may have been a bit ahead of his time when he penned those words. But the 5,000 people who responded to this survey would heartily agree.

No lazy bunch, this group. They reported a heavy reliance on physical as well as mental exercises to heal hurting bodies and soothe jangled nerves. Almost 3,800 said they tried walking to lose weight, for example.

More than 3,800 walked to relieve tension or depression, and more than 2,400 tried meditation to relieve tension or stress.

That's a positive sign, says Lyle Micheli, M.D., director of the Sports Medicine Division and associate clinical professor of orthopedic surgery at Harvard Medical School. "The physical exercises these people used—walking, swimming or aquatics, yoga and strength training—are all safe, inexpensive and easy to do."

Now these pursuits may sound more like recreation than medicine. To be sure, most people do find them enjoyable. But research has been highlighting their powerful health benefits as well.

Take the mental/emotional remedies in the survey—meditation, prayer and music, for example. "All of these therapies have one thing in common," says Herbert Benson, M.D., chief of the Division of Behavioral Medicine and president of the Mind/Body Medical Institute at New England Deaconess Hospital, Boston, and associate professor of medicine at Harvard Medical School. "They all elicit the 'relaxation response.'"

The relaxation response is the opposite of the arousal (fight-or-flight) response. During the arousal response, the hormones adrenaline and noradrenaline are released. They in turn cause an increase in metabolism, heart rate and blood pressure, research shows. They also bring about feelings of anxiety, anger and depression. But when people elicit the relaxation response, metabolism, heart rate and blood pressure calm down. If they do it regularly, they have a greater sense of peace and control.

"So to the extent that any symptom or disorder is caused or made worse by stress," says Dr. Benson, coauthor of *The Wellness Book,* "the relaxation response is useful."

Actually, scores of symptoms can be caused by stress: nausea, vomiting, diarrhea, constipation, short temper, high blood pressure and heart rhythm abnormalities, to name a few. And some symptoms, such as pain, are made worse by it.

The Power of Commitment

Now physical and mental exercises don't generally give you the kind of instant, dramatic results you might see from a "wonder" drug. But the results are often amazing if you stick with them.

Relaxation-response exercises may not reduce your anxiety as fast as tranquilizers can, but they can often be just as powerful if they're done consistently—without the powerful side effects. In the same way, walking may not eliminate backache as quickly as a painkiller, but it may be more effective in the long run.

Exercise remedies have their greatest impact when they become a regular part of your lifestyle. While they're easy to do, they do require patience and motivation because they take more effort than just taking medication. Clearly, the exercise remedies are for those who are committed to self-care and taking control.

The "good," "fair" or "poor" rating for each exercise remedy indicates those you think are overwhelming successes as well as those you probably wouldn't write home about. None were real losers, though.

The survey results shouldn't be confused with scientific evidence. They're just a report of how well people said the remedies worked for them.

Physical Exercises

Walking to Relieve Tension or Depression ▶ Walking ran away with top honors among the physical exercises included in the survey. Eighty-nine percent of those who tried this feet-first approach said they got "good" results. Another 10 percent reported "fair" results, giving walking a near-perfect track record for fighting tension and depression among the survey respondents.

"Exercise burns off the adrenaline and noradrenaline released during fight-or-flight response—the way they were meant to be burned off—by 'fleeing,'" says Dr. Benson.

Studies at California State University have shown significant reductions in tension after walking. And in another study by the Florida Department of Health and Rehabilitative Services, people in an eight-week walking program reduced the stress they felt at work by 30 percent.

"There are two basic steps necessary to elicit the relaxation response," says Dr. Benson. "First, there must be a focus, often a repetitive device such as a word, sound or thought. And second, when other thoughts intrude, they should be passively disregarded and attention brought back to the focus. With walking, you start off with your worries, but the repetitiveness of your footfall and the cadence of your breathing take over."

Studies suggest that people who are depressed feel better when they exercise regularly and that a moderate increase in aerobic capacity has a significant antidepressant effect.

Some scientists think the exercise-induced release of endorphins—brain chemicals that seem to produce a feeling of well-being—are responsible. Twenty minutes of walking three times a week is probably a minimum for having an aerobic effect.

"I have had depression problems all my life," said a respondent from Gladstone, New Jersey. "When a doctor put a label on the problem and told me it was treatable, exercise became my remedy of choice. I walk 45 minutes to one hour, six times a week. My bouts of depression are infrequent now, and when they do occur, I can handle them with great strength."

And a woman from Rogue River, Oregon, said, "I do waitress work, so I walk for a living. It's hard to judge the effects. But a walk in the country with fresh air helps my mental health and increases my stamina."

Walking to Relieve Circulatory Problems ▶

Studies show that regular walking can decrease levels of

artery-clogging blood fats while increasing the level of high-density lipoprotein (HDL), the beneficial kind of cholesterol.

Walking can also help take the pressure off varicose veins in the legs and reduce the pain of intermittent claudication, or clogged leg arteries, by promoting better circulation.

Forty-nine percent of those who answered the survey tried walking for circulatory problems. Eighty-five percent reported good results.

"Walking has greatly reduced my leg pains from varicose veins," said a woman from Newton, Massachusetts. "I try to walk about three miles, five or six days a week."

And a woman from Lyons, Michigan, said, "Walking has been a very good remedy for me. I've lost 60 pounds and reduced my cholesterol, blood pressure and stress."

Walking to Lose Weight ▶ Eighty percent of survey respondents who tried to walk off some excess weight met with success. Seventy-six percent tried this method.

"Not everyone can lose weight through exercise alone," says Dr. Micheli. "Perhaps the high success rate of the people surveyed reflects some changes in diet as well as exercise." In any case, walking is ideal: Most anybody can do it, especially if they start out slowly and equip themselves with a proper pair of shoes.

"I instruct people to do this kind of exercise by their watch," says Dr. Micheli. "Estimates of distance can be wildly inaccurate. But you can trust the clock." Be realistic and start out at a comfortable pace for a short period of time, he says. "Increase gradually—about 10 percent a week. If you're walking 20 minutes three times a week, for example, you can probably safely increase to 22 minutes three times a week."

The rate at which fat burns for any type of exercise increases after the first 20 minutes. So if you want to lose fat, walk more than 20 minutes at a time.

If you're 50 pounds overweight or more, seek a doctor's advice first. Ditto if you get chest pains during exercise or have chronic foot or leg problems.

"I can't say enough good things about walking," said

a woman from Redlands, California. "I was severely over-weight and had dieted off and on almost all my life (69 years). When I ate sensibly and walked, I lost 126 pounds. If I keep walking, I can keep the weight off, and I feel great and much happier with myself."

And a woman from Alexandria, Louisiana, said, "I walked to work for two years and went from a size 16 to a size 10 dress. And I never went on a diet. Everyone want-ed to know what kind of diet I was on. They could not believe it."

Walking to Lower Blood Pressure ▶ Thirty-four percent of those who answered the survey tried to walk their blood pressure down. Seventy-nine percent of them said they got good results. "There is some evidence that walking can help lower blood pressure in some people, but I'm surprised at how many people were aware of that," says Dr. Micheli. "That's rather sophisticated knowledge."

Some people with mild hypertension may be able to eliminate their medication or reduce the dosage with a regular walking program.

Walking seems to give your cardiovascular system a workout without raising already high blood pressure to dangerous levels, as some more aggressive types of exer-cise can. Walking also helps fight obesity, a common trig-ger for high blood pressure.

If you're taking blood pressure medication, talk with your doctor before beginning an exercise program. Set up a regular schedule of visits to monitor your program. And don't change the dosage of any of your medicines without your doctor's approval.

"I have been on a walking exercise program for three months, and it definitely improved my blood pressure reading, which has always been a big concern to me and my doctor," said a woman from Fort Dodge, Iowa.

And a woman from White Salmon, Washington, said, "I was on blood pressure pills for ten years and complete-ly eliminated them by walking, losing weight, reducing salt intake, eating a low-fat, high-fiber diet and eating garlic."

33
∎

Swimming or Aquatics to Relieve Arthritis ▸ "Swimming and water aerobics help my arthritis more than anything I have ever tried," said a woman from Hopkinsville, Kentucky.

A respondent from Wilbraham, Massachusetts, echoed that sentiment. "Swimming two to three times weekly in an indoor heated pool has definitely kept my arthritis pain from getting worse."

Water works, said the survey respondents. Seventy-seven percent of those who took to the water said they got good arthritis relief. Twenty-four percent of the 5,000 tried either swimming or aquatics, which can include walking in a pool and range-of-motion exercises.

"When I have patients who can't walk without pain, I put them in a water program and often see dramatic results," says Dr. Micheli. "They can improve their fitness without pain. And this can be the first step to other types of exercise. I also think people enjoy doing things in groups. The social aspect can help."

Aquatic exercise is an excellent way to improve and maintain joint flexibility and increase muscle strength. The water displaces body weight, easing stress on the joints. You may even feel as though the water is massaging you. And because exercising in water is less painful, people are more likely to make it a habit.

Strength Training for Greater Energy ▸ Seventy-six percent of the folks who tried strength training said it did a good job of increasing their "energy level." Twenty-five percent of the respondents tried to muscle up a bit.

"To my knowledge, no research studies have looked at this," says Ken Kontor, executive director of the National Strength and Conditioning Association, "because a person's perception of energy would be subjective and hard to quantify. But as people get stronger, they can perform everyday activities with greater ease and efficiency, and probably 'feel more energetic' as a result."

34

"In studies at Tufts University, for example, researchers found that elderly people can get dramatically stronger with rather simple exercises," says Dr.

Micheli, "and also increase their 'functional ability'—what they are able to do. I often recommend strength training for older people, who can lose muscle tone fast."

Some studies suggest that strength training may also lower your total cholesterol level while raising the level of HDL, the good cholesterol. There's also evidence it can lower your blood pressure and blood sugar levels and fight osteoporosis, the bone-thinning disease.

Now we're not talking about the kind of vein-popping, neck-bulging, beef-building activities that make a Mr. Universe out of a 97-pound weakling. We mean a kinder, gentler kind of resistance exercise aimed at building healthier bodies, not bigger ones.

Walking to Relieve Back Pain ▶ "After ten months of physical therapy for back pain to no avail, I began walking and voilà! No back pain," said one satisfied respondent. "When I stop walking, the pain returns within one to two weeks."

A respondent from Fleetwood, Pennsylvania, told a similar tale. "Two years ago I had a ruptured disk. I had surgery. The only therapy my doctor gave me was to walk as much as I could, and today I feel great."

Seventy-three percent of those who tried walking for their back pain got good results. And 47 percent of the 5,000 tried this mobile cure.

"Those are impressive figures," says Dr. Micheli. "But it makes sense. There is evidence that when you walk, your abdominal muscles become stronger and increase their endurance. The stronger your abs are, the more support they'll provide to your back."

If you have a bad back, don't undertake a walking program without a doctor's okay. Rest is usually the prescription for acute back pain. And walking can worsen problems like degenerative disk disease.

Yoga to Relieve Pain ▶ This ancient practice is often recommended by doctors in pain-control programs. Yoga's combination of breathing, relaxation and stretching exercises may constitute a triple threat to pain. And although it hasn't yet been subjected to scientific scrutiny, yoga is sufficiently safe and potentially helpful to warrant giving it a try, if you see fit.

Yoga exercises are performed slowly, without the kind of jerky motions that are more likely to cause injury. And the good posture that yoga teaches may be especially helpful for people with low back pain.

Although only 18 percent of the 5,000 survey respondents tried to relieve pain with yoga, 63 percent claimed it brought them good relief.

Mental/Emotional Remedies

Pets to Relieve Loneliness or Stress ▶ Pets beat prayer by a whisker to top the list of mental/emotional remedies in the survey. Pets boasted an 87 percent success rate for helping people defuse stress and overcome loneliness. Sixty-two percent of the 5,000 respondents said they gave a warm, fuzzy companion a try.

"I'm not surprised by these results," says Dr. Benson. "Loneliness is such a devastating feeling that companionship—be it human or animal—is very important."

Americans seem to understand this—there are more pets than children in American households! And it's not hard to see how petting a purring cat can be relaxing.

People who live alone have more heart disease than those who live with another person or a pet, studies show. Heart attack victims who have pets live longer. And elderly people with pets seem to hold up better following stressful events—they make fewer trips to the doctor, researchers found. In fact, just gazing at tropical fish may temporarily lower blood pressure.

In some situations, tail-wagging friends seem even more calming than close human friends. Women faced with stressful, mental, arithmetic tasks had lower blood pressures and pulse rates when their dogs were present than when they were alone or accompanied by a close friend.

"The presence of pet dogs...provided the kind of nonevaluative social support that is critical to buffering physiological responses to acute stress," the researchers say.

"A loving pet is truly the best medicine," said a woman from Park Forest, Illinois.

A man from Glen Burnie, Maryland, said, "Holding and petting a lap cat or small dog for reducing blood pressure and stress works for me."

And a woman from Bloomington, Minnesota, said, "Before I got married I was in an extremely high-stress executive position. My cat and his devotion were a godsend. The stress seemed to accentuate my being alone and any other problem. It was so good to have this wonderful little animal to love me and depend on me. It's such unconditional love."

Prayer to Relieve Tension or Stress ▶ Eighty-six percent of those who answered the survey attest to the tension-busting power of prayer, saying they got good results. Sixty-eight percent of the 5,000 tried this path to personal peace and quiet.

It was Dr. Benson who pioneered scientific research into the effect of prayer on stress reduction. While exploring ways to evoke the relaxation response, he taught patients a simple relaxation method: to make themselves comfortable, sit quietly and silently repeat a word or phrase.

"Eighty percent of my patients chose a word or prayer arising from their faith," says Dr. Benson, "even though they were offered the choice of other soothing words, such as *peace* or *ocean.*"

What's more, people who used words related to their own religion persisted with the program longer and enjoyed greater improvement in health. Dr. Benson coined the term *faith factor* to describe this phenomenon. "Any technique that elicits the relaxation response will work," says Dr. Benson, "but it will work better if you choose one that conforms to your belief system—something you're comfortable with." (For some people that may be prayer, and for others, meditation, biofeedback or something else.)

"Prayer has been unbelievable!" according to a woman from Bryantown, Maryland. "Going deep into prayer, thinking and praying for others and myself, too, has been wonderful, peaceful and answered!"

"Often I hesitate to end my prayer for the relaxation it brings," said a woman from Plano, Texas.

And a respondent from Butte, Montana, said, "I don't think anything can beat prayer for tension. Just ask for God's help, and then put things in His hands and leave them there. Don't keep taking them back again! It'll get you through any crisis."

Music to Relieve Tension or Stress ▶ More people said they used this method than any of the other mental/emotional remedies—77 percent. And 82 percent of them said it brought them good relief.

When music is played for patients before, during or after surgery, it seems to reduce anxiety as well as lessen pain and speed recovery, some studies found. When soothing music was played in an operating room during surgery, for example, the patients required less sedative—by half!

Some experts think it's the rhythm that helps music work its soothing magic. Others think it's the tonal qualities or just personal preference that determines whether this tranquilizer on tape—or CD or record album—does the trick.

"I use soothing instrumental music—no vocals!" said a respondent from Centerville, Utah. "I lie with my legs elevated, with a pillow and blanket, near a warm light or fireplace. Very relaxing! I use music that brings back happy times and memories."

And a woman from Fremont, California, said, "I use classical music to de-stress driving."

Touch Therapy to Relieve Tension or Stress ▶ Touch therapy is any of a number of hands-on healing techniques that deliver mental as well as physical benefits—massage being the most notable.

Thirty-two percent of those who answered the survey tried one of these techniques to melt away stress or tension. Of those, 78 percent said they got relief.

Although massage has been studied to some extent, there's precious little evidence as to exactly how it relieves stress. Doctors know that mental tension can translate into muscle tension during the arousal response—through the release of adrenaline and noradrenaline. The soothing physical sensations produced by massage or other touch therapies may feed back to the brain and reduce anxiety. The brain, in turn, tells all the muscles to relax, the theory goes. That may be why massaging one area can produce an all-over feeling of relaxation.

Whatever the mechanism, it's becoming clearer that human beings have an innate need to be touched. One study showed that premature babies who were caressed and massaged began to thrive—gaining weight almost 50 percent faster than other preemies receiving only routine holding and rocking. Their nervous systems developed faster, and they were more active and responsive than the others.

A respondent from Auburn, New York, summed it up: "My weekly massage really helped after I was widowed. It was good therapy having someone touch me after my husband passed away, and it relaxed me."

Meditation to Relieve Tension or Stress ▶ "Transcendental meditation is wonderful," said a man from New Port Richey, Florida. "I meditate twice daily. I am 87."

The meditation techniques that bring about the relaxation response are even older than that—they have their roots in Eastern religions. The technique called transcendental meditation (TM) is just one form. Science has clearly proven its stress-reducing effectiveness.

Technically, you must take a special course to learn TM. During the course, your teacher presents you with a secret "mantra," a sound to meditate on. But as Dr. Benson has found, meditation doesn't have to take the specific form of TM to be effective in evoking the relaxation response. It can be as easy as finding a quiet place, sitting up comfortably and focusing on your breathing, on a word or on an image and gently dismissing any intruding or wandering thoughts.

It's best to meditate at the same time and place every

day. And try to do it every day, if only for a minute. With practice, you can work up to a healthy 20-minute sitting.

Seventy-seven percent of those who tried meditation found they got good, calming results. Forty-nine percent of the 5,000 gave it a shot.

Visualization to Relieve Physical or Emotional Problems ▶ If you can picture it, you're more likely to be able to do it. That's the reasoning behind the use of visualization, or imaging, to overcome emotional obstacles, improve performance, ease pain or promote relaxation.

Athletes and business executives have been using this technique to improve performance for years. And one study lends some scientific credence to the practice. College students with a fear of public speaking were able to overcome their apprehension by envisioning the best possible scenario: wearing just the right clothes, feeling confident and well prepared, giving a brilliant speech that was well received. Practicing this kind of visualization worked better than some other stress-reduction techniques, such as muscle relaxation and desensitization, in this study.

By conjuring up detailed pictures of relaxing situations in your mind, you can help dissolve stress, too. To try this, lie down, close your eyes, and focus on your breath. After a few minutes, begin to imagine yourself in a relaxing scene—lying on a beach, for example. Hear the waves, smell the salty air, feel the warm sun. Picture your tension receding with the waves. For best results, listen to a tape describing the relaxing scene or have someone guide you through it.

If you're comfortable with this, it should work well for you as a way of eliciting the relaxation response, says Dr. Benson.

Of those who tried visualization in our survey, 65 percent got good results. Thirty-eight percent of the 5,000 respondents gave it a try.

"I found visualization tremendously helpful with depression and also with sticking to a diet and exercise plan. As I walk, I visualize how I want to look, and the image keeps me from temptation," said a respondent from Gladstone, New Jersey.

Biofeedback to Relieve Stress or Pain ▸ Seventeen percent of those who answered our survey said they turned to machines for help in their war on stress. Sixty-one percent of them were happy with the outcome.

A de-stressing machine? Well, sort of. Biofeedback is a method of consciously influencing bodily functions you don't ordinarily have conscious control of: blood flow, nervous muscle tension, heart rate, brain waves, even perspiration. A monitoring machine measures one or more of these functions and translates them into audio or visual cues (feedback). As you learn to control the cues, you influence the body function they reflect. If you're one who can master the technique, you're eventually able to do away with the machine and affect heart rate, and other areas, on your own.

Biofeedback appears to be a moderately effective treatment in stress-related conditions, such as tension and migraine headaches, insomnia and high blood pressure, several studies suggest.

"I do meditation relaxation and biofeedback every day for migraines," said a respondent from Shreveport, Louisiana. "I have fewer headaches and need less medicine. I now have a more 'in-charge' feeling."

A fellow respondent from Boulder, Colorado, added, "I successfully used biofeedback to reduce high blood pressure and get off medication."

Flotation Tanks to Relieve Tension or Stress ▸ You float in a large bathtub filled with pleasantly warm water (and lots of Epsom salts to increase buoyancy), encased in a sealed, soundproof container. The silence and lack of all external stimuli melt your stress away. At least, that's the theory behind the use of flotation tanks to douse tension.

Seven percent of those who took part in our survey tried to float their way to calmer nerves. Fifty-one percent of them said it did a good job.

Science has yet to fully investigate flotation tanks

and stress relief. But you may be able to achieve muscle relaxation and other stress-relieving effects with plain old warm baths, experts say. Stick with water that's comfortable—100° to 102°F. (Hot water can have the opposite effect.) Limit your soak to 15 minutes.

"We use a hot tub/spa for relaxation, pain and my arthritis," said a couple from 29 Palms, California. "It's wonderful to sit and just talk." And a woman from Bethel, Connecticut, said, "To relax and relieve that glum feeling after a rainy day, I take long soaks in a tub with Epsom salts or herbal essences."

Hypnosis to Relieve a Physical or Emotional Problem ▶ Imagine being so caught up in a good movie that you forget it's a movie, that you're in a theater or that you'll have to drive home when it's over. That's how one doctor describes the hypnotic state.

A doctor who practices hypnosis will use a variety of methods to help you relax and focus your attention. He might speak in a monotone, for example, directing your thoughts to your heavy eyelids or a serene image.

Then, depending on your reason for seeking treatment, the doctor will give you "cues," or suggestions to help. The doctor might also suggest some phrases to repeat to yourself between sessions. At the session's end you simply open your eyes, fully aware of all that transpired.

Hypnosis is often used to treat conditions that are related to stress or fear, like eating disorders, fear of flying and insomnia, although hard-core evidence of its efficacy is sparse. And it's often prescribed for people with chronic pain, to help increase their ability to tolerate it.

Of course, you can use similar techniques on your own (self-hypnosis) to help fight stress or relieve medical conditions. "If you're so inclined," says Dr. Benson, "it should be an effective technique for you to evoke the relaxation response."

And many people did try this as a home remedy. In the survey, 51 percent of those who tried hypnosis got the desired result, with 18 percent of the 5,000 giving it a chance.

And a woman from Waterbury, Connecticut, claimed, "Hot packs and hypnosis have helped greatly for my muscle tension and migraine headaches."

A Healing Potpourri 5

*Classic home remedies
from yesterday and today.*

Chances are, you learned about them from your mom. And she learned about them from her mom, and so on. No, we're not talking about the facts of life. We're talking about home remedies—the "classics" of home care.

These aren't the kind of high-tech medical miracles you might hear about on the evening news. Many of them involve the use of simple household products and have likely been in use for generations. Take the old standby, saltwater gargling, for example. Almost 4,000 of the 5,000 people who responded to the survey said they tried this method of swishing away sore throat pain.

But not all of the remedies in this varied group are as old as the hills. Others are more modern but seem destined to become classics nevertheless. Over 2,000 of the respondents to the survey said they've tried special pillows to relieve neck or back pain—a relatively newfangled invention but one that's apparently catching on quickly.

Regardless of their heritage, these types of remedies seem to have broad appeal. "They're fairly inexpensive, safe and readily available," says Ara H. DerMarderosian, Ph.D., professor of pharmacognosy and medicinal chemistry at the Philadelphia College of Pharmacy and Science. "Many people were born and brought up on these simple remedies. If they seem to work effectively, there's nothing wrong with using them for minor ills." (Of course, any serious medical problem deserves to be evaluated by a doctor.)

The key question is, Do they work for you? The survey ratings of "good," "fair" or "poor" results point out some real hot crowd pleasers, a few that did a lukewarm job and one stone-cold fish.

While the survey results don't prove whether the remedies really work or not, they do allow people to share their home-remedy experiences with fellow respondents—5,000 of them! And here's what they said.

Cold Packs
for Recent Injury or Swelling

When it comes to a painful injury, the 5,000 respondents who answered the survey said, "Ice it!" Ninety percent reported "good" results with this fresh-from-the-freezer remedy. More than 9 percent more reported "fair" results, for an almost perfect success rate and the highest score of any remedy on the survey.

Cold can constrict blood vessels to put a clamp on swelling and internal bleeding. The less blood that collects around an injury, the shorter the healing time. And cold reduces muscle spasm. All these actions have been confirmed by science and make cold therapy top-notch first aid for acute injuries like muscle strains, sprains and bruises.

"A cold pack stops my muscle pain almost instantly and lasts long enough for me to get to sleep," said a woman from New Albany, Indiana.

Of course, it's still important to elevate an injury and to see a doctor if it's serious—if it's bleeding, not getting better or not being soothed by over-the-counter pain relievers.

Depending on your cold tolerance, you can apply a rubberized ice bag or cold gel pack for 20 minutes with little danger of frostbite. (Applying ice directly to skin, though, can harm tissue.) You can repeat this every two hours. But forget this remedy if you've got a circulatory problem or if you can't feel properly for any reason.

Massage/Body Work
for Muscle Pain or Tension

When you get a crick in your neck, what's the first thing you do? Rub it? Most people do. "It seems to be a built-in mechanism," says Charles Norelli, M.D., staff physiatrist at Good Shepherd Rehabilitation Hospital in Allentown, Pennsylvania. "If a muscle is sore, you massage it."

Just because it's a reflex doesn't mean it works. But the respondents reported extraordinary success using massage to smooth away muscle pain and tension. In fact, 87 percent of those who tried it reported good results from this healing technique. Fifty-six percent said they tried this.

The most popular use of massage is for stress relief. Mental tension quickly translates into muscle tension. Massage can reverse that trend and relax you. Doctors aren't sure how. As a respondent from Gulf Breeze, Florida, put it, "Massage is a must in my life for reducing muscle tension and stress."

Massage may reduce muscle pain and fatigue after exercise by helping to remove lactic acid, a metabolic waste product that builds up in exercised muscles. And because massage stimulates circulation of both blood and lymphatic fluid (which tend to pool around the site of an injury), it can help reduce swelling and maybe even promote healing.

"Massage worked better than drugs for my husband after he injured his rotator cuff [shoulder]," said one respondent. "I use massage for arthritis pain relief and stress reduction."

And a respondent from Versailles, Kentucky, said, "Our favorite 'de-headacher' (for tension headaches) is a scalp and facial massage. It works every time!"

But note: If you have high blood pressure or other circulatory or heart problems, if you're prone to internal bleeding or blood clots or if you have a serious infection or cancer, ask your doctor first if massage is okay. Finally, don't massage near a severe muscle strain or tear within the first 72 hours, or near a suspected fracture.

Hot Packs or Water Jets for Muscle Pain

Try this remedy during the first 72 hours after an injury and you're likely to get more pain, not less! That's because heat can increase bleeding and swelling. After

45
∎

that, though, heat can work its soothing magic. It's a proven therapy—heat removes debris from an area that's been injured and brings healthy nutrients with increased circulation. Heat causes muscles to relax and allows tissues to extend a bit more, bringing greater freedom of movement.

Roughly 83 percent of respondents who tried this remedy said they got good relief. About 60 percent of those surveyed tried this.

Moist heat is best at seeping into tissues. One method is to place a wet hand towel in the microwave for a few minutes and heat it to a tolerable temperature. (It's safe if you can pick it up without discomfort.) Wrap that in a dry towel and apply to the sore spot. Or you can buy a gel pack made specifically for this purpose. Follow the manufacturer's directions. Treat at a comfortable temperature for 30 minutes, four to six times a day.

Other good methods: Apply an old-fashioned hot-water bottle or a warm, moist towel in a plastic bag. Be wary of sources of dry heat, such as electric heating pads, though. It's easy to get burned because they don't cool off—they maintain a constant heat until you turn them off. If you must use this method, don't lean or lie on the pad or fall asleep while using it. Don't combine heat with any type of ointment. And don't use heat at all if you have either of the conditions mentioned as being off-limits for cold therapy.

Finally, don't overlook the most common form of heat therapy: a warm (not hot) bath or shower. But avoid aiming forceful jets directly at the aching area—that just chases away healing blood flow. "I use a hot shower to reduce back- and neck-muscle pain and to reduce tension and stress," said a respondent from Maryville, Tennessee.

Back Support for Back Pain

Forty-five percent of the respondents who answered the survey tried using a back support in their chair or car seat. Seventy-nine percent claimed it brought them good relief from back pain.

"That's consistent with research that shows that 80

percent of back pain is 'mechanical,'" says Dr. Norelli. "That means it's related to the bones, ligaments and muscles. And they, in turn, are affected by posture. Back supports help by keeping your back in 'physiological lordosis'—its natural curve."

There's no mystery to it, says Dr. Norelli. Simply sit in a chair and put your hand behind your lower back, palm facing out, at about belt level. "That's just about enough to keep you in a good position," he says, "and take excess pressure off the disks, muscles, ligaments and bones." And that's what to look for in a back support. It should be rigid enough to hold you in that position.

These supports can help just about any kind of back problem except spinal stenosis, a narrowing of the spinal canal that can occur in older people, says Dr. Norelli. But they won't necessarily cure the problem. "Back pain can have many causes," he says. "It may be that a couple of muscles simply need to be stretched out. And learning the proper stretches would cure it. Or it could be something more serious. Either way, you don't want to keep 'putting Band-Aids' on a problem that is not getting better or is getting worse or is disabling. You should see a doctor, find out what it is and get it corrected."

With that advice in mind, though, back supports can be a big help. "I used a back-support pillow while driving on a 4,000-mile road trip," said a woman from Orange, California. "Result—no sign of my usual back pain."

Meat Tenderizer
for Insect Bites/Stings

"I tried meat tenderizer for a very painful wasp sting on my instep (I stepped on one while barefoot)," said a respondent from Chino Hills, California. "I made a paste with water, rubbed it into the sting hole—fantastic relief!"

"Some meat tenderizers contain papain, an enzyme from the papaya plant that breaks down proteins," says Dr. DerMarderosian. "That's how they make meat more tender. Papain works on insect bites by breaking down

47

proteins in the insect poisons." By inactivating some of the venom, it dissolves some of the pain. Applying it quickly may help you avoid some or all of the pain and inflammation.

About 77 percent of those who tried meat tenderizer on the zing of a sting said they got good relief. Twenty-eight percent of those who answered the survey gave this a stab.

First, check the label of your meat tenderizer to make sure it contains papain. (Some brands don't.) Gently flick out the stinger with a fingernail or file, then briefly apply ice or cold water. Apply a thin layer of paste made from tenderizer and water.

(Of course, if you're allergic to bee stings, or if you start to have a reaction—hives or difficulty breathing—get medical treatment immediately.)

Baking Soda for Insect Bites/Stings

Twice as many respondents (56 percent) tried this remedy as tried meat tenderizer. But the results were almost identical, with 76 percent reporting good results.

"The soothing qualities of baking soda [sodium bicarbonate] have been known for centuries," says Dr. DerMarderosian. "It works because a paste made with water retains moisture and produces an alkaline medium. That means it can neutralize things that are acidic, such as the irritating venom of an insect sting."

In one study, baking soda reduced the pain of local anesthetic injections by lowering the acidity of the anesthetic solution. The baking soda made the anesthetic work faster and longer to boot.

Special Pillow
for Neck or Back Pain

When life gives them a pain in the neck, some people find relief in a pillow. In the survey, 75 percent said they got good results by changing to a special neck pillow.

Forty-three percent of the respondents gave it a whirl.

"These pillows help for the same reason that back supports help," says Dr. Norelli. "They help keep your neck in a neutral position, supporting its natural curve while you sleep. That can help ease the pain of nerve, bone and muscle problems."

Most special neck pillows are contoured to support your neck when you sleep on your back or sides, and they leave a depression for your head. Look for one that's the right height for your neck curve. Too low and it won't do much good. Too high and it will hyperextend your neck.

If you sleep on your side, look for a pillow that's just thick enough to equal the distance from your ear to the outside of your shoulder, says Dr. Norelli. "If the pillow's not high enough, you can beef it up by placing a folded blanket or towel underneath. Avoid sleeping on your stomach if you have a problem with neck pain."

Again, serious problems should be seen by a doctor, with the pillow playing only second fiddle to treatment. As such, though, it can still be beneficial. "I started using a contour pillow eight years ago to relieve neck pain caused by degenerative disk disease," said a woman from Stuart, Florida. "It made a dramatic difference."

Another respondent, from Baltimore, Maryland, said, "I suffered for years with morning headache and back stiffness until I began using a special pillow." Finally, a woman from Ellenton, Florida, reported, "I am convinced of the value of the neck pillow and a special one for the small of the back to help spinal problems. Mine have kept me from surgery!"

Decongestant or Modified Valsalva Maneuver to Prevent/Relieve In-Flight Ear Pain

It can be a great relief when your plane lands safely. But not if your ears are in searing pain. Unfortunately, that's one of the discomforts of air travel for some.

The problem? As the plane descends through the atmosphere, outside air pressure increases. If your eustachian tubes are blocked, the pressure inside your ears can't follow suit, and the result is ear pain.

If you're prone to this malady, using a decongestant pill or nasal spray can be a super ear saver. "It's an excellent preventive measure," says Stanley Farb, M.D., chief of otolaryngology at Montgomery Hospital and Sacred Heart Hospital in Norristown, Pennsylvania. "Use it about one hour or so before descent. It's safe and effective for most people." Just be sure to heed package warnings.

Seventy-three percent of those who tried this said it worked well for them. Twenty-one percent of the 5,000 respondents tried to head off ear pain using this remedy.

This isn't the only weapon at your disposal, however. You can reduce pressure as you feel it building by performing a simple trick called the modified Valsalva maneuver. Hold your nostrils closed by pinching them together right near the bottom. Blow air gently into your nose so that your nose balloons out gently over your fingers. That helps open up the eustachian tubes and equalize the pressure. You can repeat this each time you feel your ears clog up.

"That's exactly what we'd do for someone who came to our office with ear pain after getting off a plane," says Dr. Farb. "This technique has been around for a long time. If you have a cold, though, blow your nose first. You want to blow air, not mucus, toward your ears."

This method brought good relief to 62 percent of those who tried it, the survey found. Thirty-four percent of the survey respondents tried to blow away ear pain this way.

Other methods that may help, too: swallowing repeatedly or yawning. "Swallowing is especially helpful for babies," says Dr. Farb. "Giving them a bottle with their favorite juice, milk or water should help."

"I always had problems with my ears when I flew," said a respondent from Arlington Heights, Illinois. "I would come home and within two days be on antibiotics for ear infections. Now when I fly, I start taking decongestants before I leave. I haven't had a problem in almost three years."

Acupressure (Shiatsu)
for Pain

Shiatsu acupressure is a form of massage based on ancient Chinese medicine. According to Shiatsu practitioners, pressure applied to specific energy pathways in the body frees up tension and the pain it can cause. While Shiatsu usually involves a practitioner who administers the "massage," people can also stimulate acupressure points themselves.

Seventy-two percent said acupressure eased their pain, with 22 percent giving this Oriental remedy a try. By comparison, 65 percent of those who tried acupuncture reported good results, with 17 percent of the 5,000 giving it a shot. (Acupuncture isn't really a home remedy but is included in the survey for the sake of comparison.)

"A hard pinch below the nose and above the lip stops a leg or foot cramp if done at the beginning of the pain," said a respondent from Silverton, Oregon. "It works 100 percent of the time for me and my husband." This trick seemed to be a favorite, with several respondents sending in similar reports.

Another popular use of acupressure among those surveyed is to prevent seasickness. Headaches also succumb to this remedy, quite a few respondents said. Just remember that Shiatsu should not be used as a substitute for proven treatments in serious illness.

Saltwater Gargle
for Sore Throat

"Salt water knocks out a sore throat faster than anything I know," said a woman from North Charleston, South Carolina.

Seventy-two percent of the people in the survey who tried it said they got good results with this simple and inexpensive remedy.

Salt water just feels soothing. And it actually does help kill germs. The higher concentration of salt in the rinse "sucks" the water out of them, giving the gargle a mild antibacterial action. It may also drain some of the excess water from swollen, inflamed throat tissues.

The solution is simple: Mix approximately ½ teaspoon of salt in eight ounces of warm water. Then gargle away. A saltwater rinse can also be used to help firm up gum tissue or treat a mouth injury.

Don't gargle if you've got laryngitis, though, as it can stress the vocal cords. And see your doctor first if you have severe, prolonged or recurrent sore throats, especially if accompanied by other symptoms.

Kegels
for Incontinence

"Even though everyone kept telling me how to do Kegel exercises, it took me the longest time to be able to do them correctly," said a respondent from Evansville, Indiana. That's why some people may be more successful with this home remedy if they have a little instruction from their doctors first.

Properly done, Kegels, or pelvic-muscle exercises, may help some people with certain types of incontinence avoid surgery or the side effects of drug therapy.

These exercises work on the slinglike group of muscles that stretch from the pubic bone in front to the tailbone in the rear. Those muscles surround the anus and urethra (the tube that drains the bladder). Squeezing them can cut off the flow—like a clamp on a hose.

Twenty-seven percent of those surveyed said they've tried Kegel exercises, with 61 percent claiming they've had good results.

"That success rate is pretty high if those people were doing it without any instruction," says Tamara Bavendam, M.D., director of female urology at the University of Washington Medical Center in Seattle. "The literature suggests that the number can be even higher than that—over 70 percent being improved or cured—when undertaken with good instruction to make sure they're exercising the correct muscles."

The research falls short of reliable scientific evidence,

however, because of the subjective nature of the record keeping. "The studies must rely on patients' reports of how often they're doing the exercises and whether they feel they're better," says Dr. Bavendam. It's not really critical, though, she says, because there's absolutely no harm in giving Kegels a try. "If they can do them correctly and they're motivated, people should benefit—both men and women."

Kegels are believed useful for patients with "stress incontinence," the loss of bladder control when they laugh, cough, run or sneeze, and "urge incontinence," the inability to hold back urine when they feel the need to go.

You can isolate the pelvic muscles on your own by turning the flow off and on when you urinate. (The same exercises can help when it comes to fecal incontinence.) While Kegeling, you can check if you're exercising the right muscles by placing your hands on your thighs and derriere. If they're contracting, you're using too many muscles.

Typically, a doctor will design a program to do at home. Usually patients are instructed to start slowly, gradually increasing the length of time they hold each contraction and the total number of contractions. A typical Kegel regimen might be 20 repetitions, each held for ten seconds, four times a day.

Some tips: "The thing I try to stress to patients is, not only are they trying to tighten the muscle, but also they need to let it relax between contractions to prevent muscle soreness," says Dr. Bavendam. "Also, it may take several weeks or months to see results. And for long-term results, they need to continue to do the exercise. It's like any muscle group—if you stop exercising it, it loses muscle strength. The good news is that most people say that once they get good results, they don't have to be as religious about the exercises as they were to achieve those results in the first place."

"Kegel exercises saved me from surgery," reported a registered nurse from Pompton Plains, New Jersey.

A woman from Croton-on-Hudson, New York, also met with success. "I really recommend the Kegel exercises," she said. "I had incontinence a while back, and due to my Kegel exercises I have eliminated it."

Brewer's Yeast
for Fleas on a Pet

Respondents were buzzing about this home remedy for sending fleas packing. "Brewer's yeast for fleas on a pet should be rated A1 Excellent!" said a respondent from Lake Oswego, Oregon.

A woman from Westmoreland, New Hampshire, reported, "Our dog is 12 years old, and we've never had a flea problem. We've always put about one tablespoon of yeast on her food. Our neighbors with pets have had some serious infestations."

Strangely, though, the survey statistics tell a somewhat different story. Twenty-seven percent of the respondents tried feeding a pet yeast as a natural flea repellent, but only 50 percent of them reported good results.

Of course, fleas can be a formidable foe even in the face of strong insecticides. And brewer's yeast is purported to be just a repellent, not a killer. (Some believe a pet exudes an odor offensive to fleas when it eats brewer's yeast.) But there have been no controlled studies showing it to be effective, says Amy Marder, V.M.D., clinical assistant professor at Tufts University School of Veterinary Medicine. "It is harmless, though."

Aspirin Used Topically
for Warts

"Aspirin on warts showed no change for me," said a respondent from Cromberg, California.

That was the prevailing sentiment, as only 35 percent of the respondents who tried this met with good results, giving this remedy the worst rating of any on the survey. (Only 6 percent of the 5,000 said they tried this.)

The remedy isn't that farfetched, however. "Aspirin is acidic," says Dr. DerMarderosian, "and acids have commonly been used to 'burn away' warts. But this probably isn't the optimum formulation, and it could cause damage to healthy skin because it's hard to know how much to use and for how long."

A closely related compound, salicylic acid, does help to peel away skin. It is the main ingredient in an over-the-counter stick-on wart patch. (Note: People with poor circulation shouldn't use these.)

To ensure the patch fits, cut out a little cardboard template exactly the shape and dimensions of your wart. Then use that template to precut a supply of patches from the adhesive plaster. Lightly coat the perimeter of the wart with petroleum jelly to prevent any of the medication from touching the skin.

Nutrition and Health Updates

Vitamins Help Erase Heart Disease

It's so simple, yet it could mean so much. One study suggests that just a single daily serving of fruits or vegetables rich in beta-carotene may reduce risk for heart attack and even stroke.

In the Nurses' Health Study of 87,245 women, groups that reported eating various amounts of beta-carotene and taking vitamin E supplements were monitored over eight years.

"We found a 22 percent reduction in the risk of heart attack and a 40 percent reduction in stroke for those women with high intakes of fruits and vegetables rich in beta-carotene compared with those with low intakes," says JoAnn E. Manson, M.D., project director for Brigham and Women's Hospital and Harvard Medical School. "We also found that high intakes of vitamin E [around 100 international units or more per day in supplement form] were associated with a 36 percent drop in heart attack risk." It isn't known whether those who took vitamin E also had healthier lifestyles that reduced risk.

Just one large carrot can provide the amount of beta-carotene that was associated with the lowest risk in this study. Other foods rich in beta-carotene that seemed to do well were sweet potatoes, mangoes, apricots, spinach and other leafy greens. Peaches, cantaloupes, broccoli, kale, papaya and yellow squash also were linked with lower risk but may require eating twice as much as the other foods, suggests Dr. Manson.

Dr. Manson says that it would be premature to recommend that women purchase beta-carotene and vitamin E supplements. However, it is reasonable to increase your intake of fruits and vegetables, she says.

Bran Beats
Breast Cancer Risk

Scientists are on their way to nailing down a surprising link between the health of women's breasts and—of all things—bran. Mounting evidence indicates that a woman's exposure to estrogen might increase her risk of breast cancer. Researchers have known for some time that women who eat a typical Western diet (high in fat, low in fiber) seem to have higher levels of estrogen in their blood than women who eat low-fat, high-fiber diets. Studies suggest that eating more fiber may help bring the risk down from the danger zone.

In one study, 62 premenopausal women were placed on diets containing 15 to 30 grams of fiber (1/2 to 1 ounce) in the form of wheat, oats or corn. Fat intake was kept constant. After two months on the wheat fiber diet, there was a significant drop in serum estrone, a type of estrogen implicated in raising cancer risk. Oat and corn fiber, however, had little effect.

In a Tufts University study, 44 healthy premenopausal women consumed diets in which both dietary fiber and fat were modulated to see what happens to estrogen levels. "Even when women were placed on high-fat diets, the high-fiber component had a positive lowering effect on the estrogen levels," says Margo N. Woods, D.Sc., assistant professor of medicine at Tufts School of Medicine. "It was the low-fat and high-fiber combination, though, that produced the most favorable benefits."

Adds David P. Rose, M.D., Ph.D., D.Sc., from the American Health Foundation, "This fits well with what we've seen in foreign countries where fat intakes are similar to ours, but their rates of cancer are much lower. It's probably related to their high fiber intake, which is why we tested fiber in the first place."

Beef Up
with Carbohydrates

Want to start building some muscle? The dinner table—not just the gym—may be one ideal place to begin. It's known that low-fat eating that's high in carbohydrates can help you lose the fat on your body without the rigors of crash dieting. One study, however, suggests a more unexpected benefit: It may also boost lean body mass—muscle.

Researchers looked at the effect on 18 premenopausal women of a high-fat diet followed for 4 weeks, then a low-fat, high-carbohydrate diet for 20 weeks. They saw an 11.3 percent decrease in fat weight. That's great—but no surprise. The 2.2 percent increase in lean body mass was the kicker. Somehow the women had generated new lean tissue without exercise!

"This is a very intriguing finding," says T. Elaine Prewitt, R.D., Dr.P.H., of the Department of Nutrition and Medical Dietetics at the University of Illinois at Chicago. "It may turn out to be yet another benefit of eating a low-fat diet."

The changes may have to do with eating more carbohydrates: The body may be less efficient at turning dietary carbohydrates into body fat than at converting dietary fat to body fat, she says. Carbohydrates also pack less of a caloric punch, carrying four calories per gram compared with nine in fat.

"The women had to eat a larger volume of food to maintain weight on the low-fat diet compared with the high-fat diet. Despite this, the women still lost weight," says Dr. Prewitt.

Just because these women got lean on dietary changes alone doesn't mean you should skip the brisk walk or the bench press. If anything, exercise adds even more to these benefits and helps maintain them over the long haul.

Potassium Pulverizes High Blood Pressure

Steering clear of a banana peel lying on the sidewalk makes perfect sense. Steering clear of a diet rich in bananas and other potassium-laden foods, however, may not—especially if you happen to be hypertensive.

Research has suggested that when potassium is subtracted from a healthy person's diet, blood pressure may rise. A preliminary study adds another cautionary twist—that people who are already hypertensive may make their blood pressure worse by depriving themselves of this important nutrient.

In this study, 12 hypertensive adults were alternately placed on a low-potassium diet and a potassium-sufficient diet. When on low potassium, their blood pressure rose significantly, with systolic pressure (the first number in a blood pressure reading) increasing seven points and diastolic (the second number) jumping by six.

"A low potassium intake may substantially increase your risk of getting hypertension or, we now suspect, may make existing high blood pressure worse," says researcher G. Gopal-Krishna, M.D., associate professor of medicine at the University of Pennsylvania. "Studies in animals and humans suggest, though, that when you get the right amount, the positive change in blood pressure may lead to a reduction in risk for stroke."

If future research confirms this, it will be even more important to add potassium-rich foods to your shopping list.

In addition, the less potassium you take in, the more calcium you may lose in your urine—stealing away an essential nutrient that helps maintain a healthy skeleton.

Exercise:
A Sex Rx

Getting your husband out of bed may help to boost his performance *in* bed. One study suggests that regular, strenuous exercise may be a potent factor in helping to boost one's sex life.

A group of 78 previously inactive but healthy men (average age 48) jogged or bicycled for an hour a day, an average of 3½ days per week, at 75 to 80 percent of their aerobic capacity. Another group of 17 men acted as a control group for comparison, not taking part in any strenuous exercise.

Nine months into the study, the more serious exercisers reported a 30 percent increase in the frequency of intercourse, with a 26 percent increase in frequency of orgasms. Other measures of arousal—caressing and passionate kissing—also were reported as increased among the exercisers. By contrast, the other men saw no improvement and actually saw slight decreases in their sexual frequency.

"The exercise may have sparked an increase in testosterone in the more active men," speculates David McWhirter, M.D., professor of psychiatry at the University of California, San Diego. According to James White, Ph.D., exercise physiologist at the University of California, San Diego, "They may also have felt better about themselves and the way they looked." Not only did their blood pressure and cholesterol drop, but also they cut their body fat by 19 percent, which may have promoted their higher self-esteem.

"Research suggests that body image and self-esteem have a lot to do with the ability to attain and maintain an erection," say the researchers. "If exercise can bolster those feelings, then it may have definite implications for nonorganic [not physically related] impotence."

Walk Off Diabetes

You've been walking up a storm. Good for you. Now walk more—try an extra mile. You won't be simply burning more calories, you may be getting something far more valuable. You may walk yourself over the threshold into full-on diabetes prevention.

"Putting a little extra oomph in your daily walk could have a real impact against development of the disease," says Susan P. Helmrich, Ph.D., an epidemiologist at the University of California, Berkeley. Dr. Helmrich has found that for every 500 calories burned during a week, risk for developing non-insulin-dependent diabetes mellitus may drop 6 percent. This 500-calorie dose translates into an extra 60 minutes of vigorous activity per week.

Dr. Helmrich reached this formula after monitoring exercise habits and future incidence of disease in 5,990 men over 14 years. Unlike other studies, researchers established the exercise patterns before disease occurred and then waited to see if and when the illness developed. "This presents a real possibility that exercise may prevent [diabetes]," says Dr. Helmrich. "We found that men who exercised regularly prevented or delayed onset of the disease."

Even more, "the most dramatic decrease in diabetes risk came in those who were most at risk for getting the disease," says Dr. Helmrich. Men who had at least one risk factor but burned 2,000 calories or more a week exercising had 41 percent less risk than those men who burned only 500 or fewer calories.

You'll hit the 2,000-calorie mark by walking three miles every day for a week. (Each mile contributes 100 calories.) Or you can fill in the gaps with comparable exercise, such as dancing, bike riding, rowing or light resistance training.

Shake the Salt, Add Some Bone

Does osteoporosis come in a bag? It's possible. Salty snacks like potato chips may end up chipping away at your bones. New research, however, suggests that by skipping the salt you may be able to prevent the calcium leak that can lead to bone loss.

In one study, researchers placed 34 postmenopausal volunteers and 25 postmenopausal patients being examined for osteoporosis on a salt-restricted diet, one week for the volunteers and two days for the patients. Urine samples were taken before and after the diets.

After the diet, the researchers found a large decrease in hydroxyproline excretion—a marker for bone destruction. According to the researchers, a reduction in sodium may allow the body to boost reabsorption of calcium, lower excretion of hydroxyproline and by implication reduce bone loss.

"If you can control the salt intake and decrease the rate of bone loss, then this has important implications for the prevention and treatment of osteoporosis," says B. Lawrence Riggs, M.D., president of the National Osteoporosis Foundation at the Mayo Clinic in Rochester, Minnesota. "But this is still experimental, and actual bone needs to be measured to see if this really works."

Skipping the salt may stop bone loss by plugging up a calcium leak from the kidney—cementing over a potential bone drain. "Some people would argue that bone loss is independent of the kidney leak, though these data suggest otherwise," says Dr. Riggs.

Fight Cholesterol with Fiber

Talk about an ounce of prevention! Now for the first time, researchers have zeroed in on how much (or how little) oat bran and oatmeal it takes to send the bad cholesterol, LDL (low-density lipoprotein), packing.

After being placed on a low-fat, low-cholesterol diet, 148 adults with high cholesterol were given oat bran, oatmeal or a non-water-soluble fiber (used as a placebo) in varying amounts every day for six weeks.

The most potent dose turned out to be either two ounces of oat bran or three ounces of oatmeal—lowering LDL cholesterol on average 10 to 15 percent. A third of those who would have required lipid-lowering drugs responded well enough to skip the pharmacy. Increasing fiber intake beyond those few ounces offered no extra reduction. The placebo had no effect.

"You don't need a whole lot to see a significant reduction—a medium-size bowl of bran or a large bowl of oatmeal did the job," says Michael H. Davidson, M.D., medical director of the Chicago Center for Clinical Research of Rush Presbyterian–St. Luke's Medical Center in Illinois. "But remember, the oat bran and oatmeal were served along with a low-fat, low-cholesterol diet—so it won't do any good to sprinkle some oat bran on your bacon and eggs and expect great results."

And remember, it takes a commitment to conquer cholesterol. "Once these people stopped eating the oat bran or oatmeal, their cholesterol levels went back up to where they were before. You need to eat it on a daily basis to maintain the reductions," he says.

Carrots Quell Cancer

Quit smoking and you've already found the best way to dramatically cut the risk for laryngeal cancer. But another line of defense against this disease may be drawn at the dinner plate.

By cutting down on fat and enlisting the help of nature's very own ground troops—broccoli, carrots and other carotenoid-rich vegetables—you may bolster your protection against laryngeal and other types of cancer.

In one study, risk for laryngeal cancer was twice as great in men with low intakes of carotenoids compared with those with high intakes. Risk was also $2\frac{1}{2}$ times greater in those with the highest fat intakes compared with those with the lowest fat intakes. These numbers were taken from research looking at the diets of 250 men diagnosed with laryngeal cancer compared with the same number of men without it. Other studies have also suggested that carotenoids may have a protective effect against laryngeal cancer.

"When we looked at vegetables individually, we didn't see anything that striking," says Jo L. Freudenheim, Ph.D., a registered dietitian and assistant professor at the State University of New York at Buffalo. "But when we looked at the carotenoid-rich vegetables as a group, they seemed to be protective."

Carotenoids are antioxidants, which may help protect against cellular damage caused by free radicals, says Dr. Freudenheim. "It's speculative, but it may be that certain types of fat encourage production of these free radicals, too," she says. That's why subtracting fat and adding vegetables and fruits is the prudent course. It may offer double doses of cancer protection.

Magnesium Wears Out Fatigue

Chronic fatigue syndrome (CFS) defies categorization and confuses doctors as easily as it devastates patients. However, researchers may have found a potentially effective treatment: injections of magnesium sulfate.

In one study, researchers compared magnesium blood levels of 20 CFS patients with those of 20 healthy people. They found all the CFS patients had lower magnesium concentrations. This led researchers to try magnesium sulfate injections.

Once a week for six weeks they gave 32 CFS sufferers either an injection of magnesium sulfate or a placebo injection. After six weeks, 12 of the 15 treated with magnesium experienced significant improvements in energy levels and emotional states. They hurt less and were able to sleep better, too. All this improvement occurred as their magnesium blood levels returned to normal. By contrast, only 3 of the 17 patients given the placebo said they felt any better.

"As of yet, we don't know how long the benefits will last—we're in the process of finding that out," says study author M. J. Campbell, Ph.D., senior lecturer at the University of Southampton General Hospital in the United Kingdom. "It may be worthwhile," says Dr. Campbell, "to check for magnesium deficiency in the blood—and if it's there, take the proper steps to fix it."

"This is an intriguing finding, but it needs to be confirmed by further studies," says Nelson Gantz, M.D., professor of medicine and specialist in infectious disease at the University of Massachusetts Medical Center and a top CFS researcher. "And remember, the magnesium sulfate was injected—it's doubtful oral supplements will have the same effect." And according to both doctors, too much oral magnesium can cause diarrhea.

Biotin for
Tougher Nails

For years no one has been able to put a finger on a potentially effective treatment for brittle nails. Now, finally, someone has—it's a little-known B vitamin called biotin. You could say the idea came straight from the horse's hoof.

After seeing how veterinarians used this water-soluble vitamin to work wonders for horses with problem hooves, Swiss researchers decided to try it out on people with brittle fingernails. In a controlled study of 32 men and women, the researchers gave one group with thin, frail and split nails six to nine months of daily treatment (2.5 milligrams, which averages 12.5 times the average daily intake). The subjects' nail thickness was boosted by 25 percent.

"Biotin is absorbed into the matrix of the nail, where it may encourage a better, thicker nail to grow," says Richard K. Scher, M.D., head of the Nail Section at Columbia Presbyterian Medical Center in New York City, commenting on the study. Dr. Scher is currently treating his brittle-nail patients with biotin supplements.

Top dietary sources of biotin are cauliflower, soybean flour, lentils, milk and peanut butter.

If you do have painful, brittle nails, see a dermatologist before doing anything on your own—they may be a symptom of something else. "It's best to let the doctor decide whether supplements are in order," says Dr. Scher. There is no current Recommended Dietary Allowance for biotin, but the amounts used in the study are believed safe.

Barley Corks High Cholesterol

Barley, an ingredient used in brewing beer, is being tapped by researchers to put a cork in high cholesterol.

When men with danger-zone cholesterol levels were given supplements of either barley flour or its oil extract, they saw their total cholesterol levels drop over 7 percent. LDL (low-density lipoprotein) cholesterol—the bad kind—dropped 9.2 percent in the oil group and 6.5 percent in the flour group. Barley flour, though, did lower HDL (high-density lipoprotein) cholesterol (the good kind) significantly, while its oil had no significant effect. By comparison, men receiving plain cellulose fiber saw no change in their cholesterol profile.

The researchers think it's the oil in the flour that's at the helm of the artery plow. "It contains tocotrienols—which are similar in structure to vitamin E," says Joanne Lupton, Ph.D., chair of the graduate faculty of nutrition at Texas A & M University. "It's this component that may be responsible for lowering cholesterol."

Low-Fat Milk
Lowers Cancer Risk

If there's a white knight of lower cancer risk, it may be low-fat milk. By switching from whole milk to a low-fat variety, you may significantly reduce your risk for ovarian cancer, suggests one study sponsored by the American Cancer Society. This kind of cancer is rare but can be deadly.

When researchers looked at milk consumption of women with and without ovarian cancer, they found that those who drank more than one glass of whole milk a day were three times more likely to have this type of cancer than those who never drank whole milk. Those who drank 2 percent milk and skim milk, though, showed a reduced risk—lower than that of people who drank no milk at all.

"This adds to the suspicion that it may be the animal fat in the whole milk that's boosting the risk," says Curtis J. Mettlin, Ph.D., chief of epidemiologic research at Roswell Park Memorial Institute in Buffalo, New York. "Why low-fat and skim milk may lower risk isn't certain, but it may be that people who drink it also have a preference for lower fats in the rest of their diet," he says.

Plus, milk houses nutrients—calcium, riboflavin and vitamins A and C—that have all been linked to reducing risk for several cancers. Consuming lower-fat milk may slice the risk of five cancers—oral, stomach, rectal, lung and cervical. Risk for these cancers rise as the intake of milk fat increases.

To switch from whole to skim milk—simply mix it up. Combine a carton of whole milk with 2 percent milk. Try that for a few weeks, then slowly reduce the amount of whole milk until you're used to 2 percent. Then introduce skim into the 2 percent. Repeat the process, phasing out the low-fat until you're happy with skim's flavor.

Salmon Salvages Heart Health

It may not be oat bran with gills, exactly, but research suggests that a diet rich in salmon may keep your good cholesterol in the swim.

After feasting on broiled salmon with dill, baked salmon, salmon salad or salmon lasagna for lunch and dinner for 40 days, a group of nine men saw one type of beneficial HDL (high-density lipoprotein) cholesterol in their blood jump an average of 10 percent.

"This particular HDL compound has been closely linked to protecting against heart attacks and heart disease," says Gary J. Nelson, Ph.D., of the U.S. Department of Agriculture's Western Human Nutrition Research Center in San Francisco. "It's usually low in men but high in premenopausal women, who tend to have lower rates of heart disease."

At the start of this study, the otherwise healthy men had below-average levels of HDL. The men's total HDL cholesterol went up in a similar fashion, while total LDL (low-density lipoprotein) cholesterol, the bad stuff, remained the same.

The mechanism behind the possible heart-healthy benefits of salmon is unclear, though one factor that might be responsible is the fact that salmon is rich in omega-3 fatty acids. When the men switched to a diet without salmon (or any other food containing omega-3 fatty acids), the effect disappeared. "These acids in the fish may help block the production of VLDL [very-low-density lipoprotein, a bad cholesterol] in the liver," says Dr. Nelson. "This may help to raise the levels of HDL, the good cholesterol."

Yogurt for Young Tummies

Some tangy yogurt may be all it takes to curb diarrhea among the diaper crowd.

When babies with diarrhea had milk replaced with yogurt in their normal diet, 86 percent saw the distress stop within five days. Among the kids fed milk instead of yogurt, only 58 percent were relieved. These results came from a study of 76 children, ages 3 to 36 months old.

"Yogurt's live cultures of beneficial bacteria can help by restoring the natural flora of the digestive system," says Pennsylvania State University food scientist Manfred Kroger, Ph.D., commenting on the study. Yogurt has been shown to roll back diarrhea among adults, he says, but this is a first for infants.

"Luckily, most babies' taste buds aren't sophisticated enough to tell the difference between yogurt and milk. But if your tot turns up her nose, try sweetening the yogurt a bit (just don't use honey for kids under a year old)," he says.

You can liquefy yogurt just by shaking it. Then it can be poured into a baby bottle. "If you use a nipple with a bigger hole, the baby can suck it out easily," says Dr. Kroger.

You should always consult your pediatrician before changing your infant's diet, however.

Carotenoids Clobber Cataracts

You may find top-notch eye protection not only in a goggle factory but in your nearby produce section as well. Researchers have just found that eating vitamin-rich fruits and vegetables is linked to lower risk of one of the "inevitables" of aging—cataracts.

In a U.S. Department of Agriculture (USDA) study, people who reported eating fewer than 1½ servings of fruit or less than 2 servings of vegetables a day were 3½ times more likely to develop lens-clouding cataracts than those who said they ate more. And people whose combined intake of fruits and vegetables was less than 3½ servings were nearly 6 times more likely to develop cataracts. The study focused on the diets of 112 people with and without cataracts.

"As you grow older, your risk for developing cataracts grows larger and larger," says Paul F. Jacques, Sc.D., an epidemiologist with the USDA Human Nutrition Research Center on Aging at Tufts University. (Studies report that cataracts may cloud the vision of up to half of all Americans over the age of 75.) "Eating a healthy diet may delay the usual aging of the lens and so delay cataracts."

How? Dr. Jacques thinks it may be due to a nutrient combo abundant in fruits and vegetables. "In other studies, we've found a pretty good link between carotenoids, vitamin C and lower cataract risk," he says. "For instance, carotenoids such as vitamin E may be key." As powerful antioxidants, they help fight oxidation, a damaging chemical reaction that may lead to cataracts.

Other research supports that theory. A Canadian study, for instance, found a lower risk of cataracts among people who got more of antioxidant vitamins C and E.

Eating
for a
Healthier Life

Vitamins plus Blood Vessels Equals Victory   6

Studies suggest vitamin C, vitamin E and beta-carotene can fight heart attacks by helping to keep blood vessels fat-free.

Mounting scientific evidence suggests the possibility that antioxidants, particularly vitamins C and E and beta-carotene, could be this decade's superheroes in the crusade to prevent heart disease.

Antioxidants "might give us new ways to deal with heart disease, over and above lowering cholesterol," says Daniel Steinberg, M.D., professor of medicine at the University of California, San Diego. He's the brains behind the "free-radical theory of atherosclerosis," what many researchers say is the best to-date explanation of the origin of heart disease and the cause of much excitement and a flurry of research in the antioxidant area.

And if preliminary results from early test-tube and animal studies are confirmed in clinical research, we might not have to look much farther than our own pantries and vegetable crispers to get the antioxidants' benefits. Increasing our intake of fruits, whole grains and vegetables may be just as important as decreasing dietary fat when it comes to heart health, says Ishwarial Jialal, M.D., assistant professor of clinical nutrition and internal medicine at the University of Texas Southwestern Medical Center.

The case for antioxidants is still theoretical and largely circumstantial at this point. But the scientific and medical communities are staking high hopes on it. If clinical trials verify what's been found under the microscope, says Dr. Jialal, "the number of deaths from heart disease in the United States and in the world will probably drop. But we can't exclude the treatment of established risk factors, like high blood pressure, cigarette smoking, high cholesterol and diabetes."

Beyond Cholesterol

The theory at the heart of all this excitement attempts to explain how heart disease starts as a minuscule spot on the artery wall and can lead to, in many people, a massive coronary. Researchers have been getting closer and closer to understanding the disease for years, making phenomenal headway when they established the link to blood cholesterol levels and dietary fat in the late 1970s. That discovery, backed by strong scientific studies, allowed them to link heart disease to high levels of cholesterol.

But most of the people who have heart attacks don't have outrageously inflated cholesterol levels. In fact, some of them are below the 200 range (the National Cholesterol Education Project recommends a level of 200 or less). And there are people who do have high cholesterol counts who have no sign of heart disease. So researchers suspect that there's more to heart disease than cholesterol alone.

Scientific research has long hinted that this "something more" may involve vitamin antioxidants. Heart attack victims have consistently low levels of vitamin C in their blood, as do smokers, who are at higher risk for atherosclerosis. Researchers have found significantly lower vitamin E levels in men with angina (chest pain that signals heart disease) than in those who were symptom-free, regardless of other risk factors, like cigarette smoking, high cholesterol and blood pressure and excess weight. Another study suggested that low vitamin E levels might have an even stronger link to heart disease deaths than well-established risk factors like high cholesterol and blood pressure.

A New Foe: Free Radicals?

So scientists set out to discover the possible connection between antioxidants, cholesterol and heart disease. Their priority was to figure out how cholesterol, specifically LDL (low-density lipoprotein) cholesterol (the worst type), gets into the walls of arteries and turns into the stuff that clogs arteries. This stuff, the fatty streaks that eventually become the advanced lesions that bypass surgery must remove, is the first sign of what could be a heart attack-to-come.

Researchers knew that the artery-blocking fatty streaks form when white blood cells enter the artery wall and there gobble up LDL. But when they paired white blood cells with LDL particles in test tubes, the white blood cells were slow to swallow the LDL. So, the researchers guessed, something must happen to LDL to make it more appetizing.

Dr. Steinberg's theory says that free radicals are the answer. Free radicals are naturally occurring, highly unstable oxygen molecules that have been accused of contributing to everything from cancer to cataracts. Their mean trick is to damage, or oxidize, body tissues and blood fats.

The effect of free radicals on LDL is similar to what happens to a steak when it sits out on the kitchen counter for too long—it goes bad. That, researchers speculate, sets off the deadly process. The white blood cells—immune cells that are out to consume their enemies—gorge themselves on the "bad stuff gone bad," thinking they're protecting the body, when they may actually be harming it. LDL-bloated white blood cells in the artery wall soon become a bulge that threatens to completely block the artery.

Fighting Back
with Vitamins

If the creation of free radicals, as scientists believe, is a naturally occurring, constant process, does that mean we're doomed to a life of congested arteries and crippling angina?

Enter the antioxidants—vitamins and enzymes in our bodies that fight oxidation caused by free radicals. Scientists believe that antioxidants may be able to stop free radicals from making LDL "go bad."

Dr. Steinberg first observed the antioxidant effect in

heart-diseased laboratory rabbits by feeding them a synthetic drug, probucol, that doctors sometimes prescribe to lower cholesterol. Dr. Steinberg's experiments revealed that the compound is also a powerful antioxidant.

And while it didn't do much to drop the rabbits' cholesterol levels, it did make a dramatic reduction in atherosclerosis, possibly because it was able to fend off free radicals. But researchers are looking into whether the natural self-sacrificing antioxidants in our food can have the same impact as antioxidant drugs on heart disease—without side effects. Most of their attention is focused on vitamin C (present in the water components of blood), the vitamin A precursor beta-carotene and vitamin E (both found in the fat components of blood, such as the LDL molecule).

Test-tube studies suggest that vitamin C may be the most potent of them all. Balz Frei, Ph.D., assistant professor of nutrition at the Harvard School of Public Health, exposed plasma to different sources of free radicals to see which of the innate antioxidants worked best. In every case, vitamin C was the first to be oxidized, indicating that it's the most protective.

"We think vitamin C traps free radicals in the surrounding environment before they can attack the LDL particle," Dr. Frei says. "And as long as there is vitamin C, free radicals cannot attack LDL because the C forms a very tight, protective shield around it."

The problem is, the vitamin C in our bodies can't keep the free radicals at bay forever. Eventually, they may consume the vitamin completely and attack the vulnerable LDL particle.

For example, during the first phase of Dr. Frei's experiments, vitamin C protected the LDL completely against detectable free-radical damage. Then, when the store of vitamin C was depleted, the antioxidants inside the LDL, like vitamin E, went to work. But E and other antioxidants inside the LDL particle were not as effective as vitamin C in blocking free radicals—some of them were able to sneak through.

By experiment's end, about one-third of the free radicals broke through the antioxidants' defense and began converting the LDL into its rancid, artery-clogging form.

In similar laboratory experiments, C has continued to outperform the other antioxidants. Dr. Jialal and his colleagues compared the reactions of vitamins C and E under stress caused by free radicals. After 24 hours of stress, vitamin C was still able to prevent almost all of the free radicals from getting to the LDL. Vitamin E had begun to give way, stopping only about 40 percent of oxidation. In a further study, Dr. Jialal showed that vitamin C was as potent as probucol in blocking LDL oxidation.

Answers to Come

It's obvious that the studies done to date, exciting though they are, have produced more questions than answers. "So far, the theory has withstood the tests it has been put to," Dr. Steinberg says. "But I want to be crystal clear that no theory is proved until there has been a very careful, very large clinical trial under the right circumstances with good controls—and that hasn't been done yet."

The first large-scale trial specifically studying beta-carotene won't be completed until late 1995 or early 1996. Researchers at Harvard Medical School are testing beta-carotene's preventive effect in the more than 21,000 heart disease–free doctors who are participating in the Physicians' Health Study. The lead researcher, Charles Hennekens, M.D., Dr.P.H., professor of medicine, professor of preventive medicine and acting chairman of the Department of Preventive Medicine at Harvard Medical School, originally set out to look at whether beta-carotene affects the incidence of cancer. Since 1984, the study participants—all men—have been taking either one 50-milligram dose of beta-carotene every other day (that's equal to two cups of cooked carrots) or a placebo pill.

But the Harvard team decided to look further into the nutrient's connection to heart disease when preliminary results suggested that beta-carotene may slow down or reverse heart disease. Over 300 men, a subgroup of the Physicians' Study, already had some sign of heart disease, unlike the rest of the study participants. After six years on the every-other-day beta-carotene regimen, 165 of these men had half as many strokes, heart attacks, cardiac deaths and artery-opening medical procedures as the 173 men on a placebo pill.

More Detective Work

The test runs in test tubes, studies on rabbits and circumstantial clues have already widened the focus of research. Dr. Jialal, for example, is currently exploring whether diabetic patients' LDL cholesterol is, for some genetic reason, even more susceptible to attack by free radicals. That would help explain why people with diabetes are at higher risk for heart disease. Other studies are looking at people with relatively low or normal cholesterol levels who develop heart disease or have heart attacks. They may oxidize LDL differently from other people, which may give doctors new ways to treat them.

Possible links between high HDL (high-density lipoprotein) cholesterol—the good stuff—and high vitamin C levels are also being studied by researchers. Studies have shown that people with higher vitamin C levels also have higher HDL levels. Paul Jacques, Sc.D., an epidemiologist with the U.S. Department of Agriculture Human Nutrition Research Center on Aging at Tufts University, speculates that vitamin C may make the already resilient HDL particle even more resistant to free-radical damage. There's also a suspected relationship between low vitamin C levels and high blood pressure.

Another spin on the free-radical theory suggests that olive oil and canola oil—predominantly monounsaturated fats—may also work as antioxidants. (Monos have already been linked to cholesterol-lowering effects, independent of their possible antioxidant role.) LDL contains both polyunsaturated and monounsaturated fats, but the free radicals have more of a taste for the polys. In a highly preliminary animal study, Dr. Steinberg found that the LDL particles of laboratory rabbits on a mono-only diet were able to better defend themselves against free radicals than the LDL of rabbits on the poly-only diet.

Rx: Eat Right

What does this mean for us, now? For one thing, the possibility that antioxidant vitamins might prevent heart disease doesn't give us license to consume mass quantities of fat-laden foods. "Lowering blood-cholesterol levels is still the primary and only proven way to reduce risk (of heart disease)," Dr. Steinberg says. "So far, we know only that antioxidants work in experimental animals, and that's not a basis for telling everybody what foods to buy and what to eat."

If the theory turns out to be a fact, keeping the fat out of our diet may leave fewer LDL particles for the free radicals to prey on.

"It would be a great tragedy if people started eating carrots and green, leafy vegetables and continued to smoke or eat high-fat foods, didn't get their blood pressure under control or remained obese," Dr. Hennekens says.

The experts say the best prescription right now is to make sure you eat enough foods containing vitamins C and E and beta-carotene—which means fruits and vegetables. The current recommendation from the National Research Council calls for five servings a day of fruits and vegetables.

This strategy would be sound even if the antioxidant theory of heart disease didn't hold up. After all, we already know that diets low in fat and rich in fruits and vegetables are linked to lower risks of heart disease and cancer. So you can't go wrong with such foods.

What about vitamin pills? "It's too early to be able to recommend to anybody whether they should or should not take supplemental vitamins, and how much," Dr. Steinberg says.

But many experts do suggest that the current Recommended Dietary Allowances for vitamins C and E might be too low and that beta-carotene may need to be added.

Good Sources
of Antioxidant Vitamins

Food	Serving	Nutrient Amount (mg)
Vitamin C		
Broccoli, fresh, boiled	1 cup	116
Cantaloupe	½	113
Orange juice, fresh	8 ounces	113
Brussels sprouts, fresh, boiled	1 cup	97
Cranberry juice	8 ounces	97
Beta-Carotene		
Sweet potatoes, boiled, mashed	1 cup	34
Pumpkin, canned	1 cup	32
Carrot, raw	1	12
Spinach, frozen, boiled	1 cup	10
Butternut squash, baked	1 cup	9
Vitamin E *(as alpha-tocopherol)*		
Sunflower seeds, dried	¼ cup	18
Sweet potatoes, boiled, mashed	1 cup	15
Kale, fresh, boiled	1 cup	10
Yams, boiled or baked	1 cup	6
Spinach, frozen, boiled	1 cup	4

Fill Up on   7
Cancer Prevention

*Researchers have found some everyday
foods have powerful potential.*

Eat your fruits and veggies and you can decrease
your chances of getting certain kinds of cancer. The
National Cancer Institute (NCI) has launched the
Designer Foods Research Project with one aim in mind:
to hunt down nutrients known as phytochemicals locked
inside common fruits, vegetables and other edible plants
(like herbs, grains and spices) and find some way to concentrate these natural cancer preventers into new
foods—superfoods with super potential.

When they've completed their work, the NCI researchers may very well have in their hands the future's
first cancer-prevention menu—a full-blown attempt to stop
the disease before it starts. Here's the strategy.

1. Identify the most powerful cancer-fighting substances
found in fruits, vegetables, herbs and other edible plants.

2. Calculate their ideal concentrations and most potent
forms.

3. Then test them in controlled trials with high-risk or
cancer patients to see if they really can stop the disease.

The mission is to stamp out the unpredictable. "Foods
are complex substances," says Herbert Pierson, Ph.D., an
NCI toxicologist and director of the five-year study. "A
food grown in one part of the country may have significant chemical differences from the same food grown in a
different location. How it's then extracted, processed or
prepared also plays a big role."

Because of these inconsistencies in composition, it's
difficult to determine how a fruit or vegetable may affect
someone's health, he says. The cancer-fighting nutrients
targeted in this program, however, would be engineered
into their purest and most powerful form—approaching

the same beneficial consistency of a mass-produced, heavily researched therapeutic substance. Newly designed, they may become edible medical missiles aimed at preventing cancer.

Diets by Design

Phytochemicals are simply chemicals found in plants that may protect them against stresses (like being eaten by animals), climate and infection. Some vitamins and many organic molecules are collectively referred to as phytochemicals. Researchers think their protective power may not be limited to just plants, however—humans may have something to gain from them, too.

"We're going after common foods plus some ingredients that people don't know much about but have been eating for years," says Dr. Pierson. "Human safety and potential anticancer activity are the major criteria."

Right now the Designer Foods Research Project is in the diaper stage—researchers are busy trying to find and fingerprint the phytochemicals while attempting to understand how they work and if they have anticancer properties. The territory's fresh, but the NCI researchers believe these nutrients may help armor the body against cancer through three mechanisms.

■ By blocking E_2 prostaglandin's tumor-promoting power. This prostaglandin is one of a group of fatty acids that performs a variety of hormonelike actions in the body. "Even though this prostaglandin is essential for the body, somehow it gets deregulated, becomes harmful and gathers in cancerous tissues," says Dr. Pierson.

■ By shunting estradiol, which is the major estrogen in a woman's body, away from tissues at risk like the breast and uterus. "When estradiol is activated, it, too, can act as a tumor promoter," says Dr. Pierson.

84

■ By hastening detoxification of certain foreign, harmful chemicals so they leave the body faster.

The Food 'Phyters

The NCI will look at an array of familiar foods—and the not-so-familiar substances inside them. Some sport names that could unravel a spelling-bee judge. Here's a quick rundown on some of these key players on the NCI Designer Foods Research Project lineup.

Garlic ▶ Evidence concerning garlic's anticancer benefits in people is preliminary but has been mounting steadily. One study found much lower stomach cancer rates in people with high garlic consumption. Another reported high consumption of garlic as being linked to lower incidence of colorectal cancer.

How might this odoriferous little package play a role in all this? Take a whiff of the stuff and you've already hit on a clue. The sulfur-containing substances that give garlic its pungent, elevator-clearing aroma are also what give it its anticarcinogenic activity.

"Research in mammals suggests that the sulfur compounds in garlic can inhibit prostaglandin metabolism," says Dr. Pierson. "They may also enhance parts of our immune system and intercept carcinogens when they're activated in our body, preventing them from damaging our cells."

Creating the right recipe that highlights the most powerful phytochemicals in garlic will take time, though. "The actions of these compounds may depend on how the garlic's prepared," says Dr. Pierson. "Raw garlic would contain a compound that does one thing, while garlic sautéed in a spaghetti sauce would contain another compound that does something else."

Flaxseed ▶ Inside flaxseed lurk two major classes of compounds that have been linked to cancer-preventive activity. One is the lignans, a type of fiber that may interfere with potentially dangerous estrogen activity on tissues vulnerable to cancer.

"Reports indicate that women who are vegetarians most of their lives have the lowest rates of breast cancer," says Dr. Pierson. "The high urinary lignan levels in vegetarians are thought to be derived from their fruit-and-vegetable diets. Research indicates that lignan levels in people who eat flaxseed approach those of vegetarians."

Further research will help determine if the key anti-cancer factor in the vegetarian diet is low-fat food intake (which has been linked to lower breast cancer risk) or substances like lignans or other phytochemicals. Several types of lignans from other medicinal plants have been used in cancer chemotherapy, he says. Flaxseed is rich in alphalinolenic acid, one of the omega-3 fatty acids. "It's essentially a plant version of fish oil," says Dr. Pierson. "Research suggests it may block the action of cancer-promoting prostaglandins."

And in Canadian studies done in animals, certain kinds of flaxseed have been shown to significantly block breast and colon carcinogens.

Licorice ▶ The licorice the NCI is chewing on isn't the candy-store kind (which is related to parsley) but rather the root originating from the legume family. Preliminary test-tube research suggests that one class of phytochemicals called triterpenoids, along with other compounds, may stifle quick-growing cancer cells, block prostaglandin production and cause some precancerous cells to return to normal growth—in a sense heading cancer off at the pass. "It may also help regulate the way we detoxify and get rid of foreign materials from our body," says Dr. Pierson.

Citrus ▶ "Chemically speaking, citrus stands out as a rich source of natural products that have been indicated as cancer preventives in much of the literature," says Dr. Pierson.

To track this wide and somewhat woolly spectrum of chemicals inside citrus fruits, Dr. Pierson is prepared to conduct basic research on how the phytochemicals are absorbed into the blood and how they might affect metabolism in humans. "The beauty of citrus, however, is that several classes of phytochemicals are highly likely to act more powerfully when they are present as a natural mixture than when they appear separately," he says.

Research may evolve around different blends of citrus fruits developed into a combination food, which will then be tested in a clinical trial.

Some of the phytochemicals Dr. Pierson is looking at include flavonoids and carotenoids, found in citrus fruits. "Both help to protect cells in the body because as antioxidants they help fight free radicals," he says. Free radicals are destructive oxygen molecules formed in the body by anything from body processes and infections to cigarette smoke and pollution. Beta-carotene and vitamin C, both free-radical-quenching antioxidants, are linked to cancer-preventive activity. Other phytochemicals found in citrus, called terpenes, may also help head off cancer-causing agents, suggests Dr. Pierson.

Cruciferous Vegetables ▸ These contain indoles and include cabbage, broccoli and kale. Indoles may inactivate tumor-causing estrogen that targets the breast. And in animal tissues, they've been shown to switch on enzymes that prevent exposure to carcinogens.

Umbelliferous Vegetables ▸ The key cancer fighters here might include celery, parsley, parsnips and beta-carotene-rich carrots. "We're interested in these vegetables because they contain a great variety of phytochemicals," says Dr. Pierson. "To harness anticarcinogenic activity, a combination of these vegetables would probably work best."

Soy ▸ "Soybeans contain compounds called isoflavones, which have a natural affinity for inhibiting an enzyme that gets overproduced in precancerous stages," says Dr. Pierson. "Soybeans are also extremely rich in other phytochemicals that may have anticancer properties."

Green Tea ▸ "Many constituents in green tea are capable of blocking cell mutations," says Dr. Pierson. "The Japanese, by drinking three to five cups a day, deliver a gram of flavonoids into their bodies each day." The green-tea flavonoids have demonstrated significant cancer-preventive activity in laboratory animal models of human cancer. Evidence suggests the dietary habit of routinely drinking green tea may be one factor linked to a decreasing incidence of gastrointestinal cancer in Japan, he says. The tea also contains a wide variety of other antioxidants.

Today's Diet, Tomorrow's Drug

According to Dr. Pierson, it's too soon to expect doctors to write out prescription recipes straight from the produce section. None of the phytochemicals under investigation has yet been shown to block the formation of cancer in humans. "But once we arrive at initial conclusions, it might be possible to target people at risk for breast, uterine, colon and perhaps even lung cancer for more detailed studies."

Until then, you shouldn't put off helping yourself to the arsenal of potential disease-fighting weapons at the grocery store. And in a few years, it may be second nature to pick up a bottle of carrot juice chock-full of cancer-beating nutrients and phytochemicals.

Says Dr. Pierson, "Isn't it time for us to protect ourselves as we develop from youth to old age? This program is the first step in that direction."

8 Delicious Results from *Prevention*'s Low-Fat Cook-Off

Some talented chefs share their best-tasting recipes.

The staff at the *Prevention* Food Center faced the formidable—though decidedly delicious—task of selecting just 12 winners from over 10,000 entries in *Prevention*

Magazine's first annual Cooking for Health Recipe Contest. After weeks of testing and tasting, the finalists were submitted for nutritional analysis. That was necessary to ensure that all conformed with the strict guidelines for fat, cholesterol and sodium content. And indeed they did! The average fat content in the winning recipes is a lean 19 percent of calories. So, without further ado—the champions!

Uncle Ben's Rice

FIRST PRIZE. Melani Juhl-Chandler, Palo Alto, California, for her Vibrant Rice and Chicken Soup.

Our testers loved this soup. "It tastes great, it looks great, and it's great for you. This dish is what our contest is all about," one judge commented. Coriander, tomato, lime juice and cayenne give Melani's soup its distinctively Mexican flavor. Add avocado and low-fat cheese and you have a fiesta of flavors and textures in every spoonful.

"I became interested in Mexican cooking after visiting the country several years ago," says Melani. "The soup is such a unique blend of tastes, it's become one of my favorite dishes." And with just 24 percent of calories from fat, it's as good for her conscience as it is for her palate.

Although Melani and her husband are quite healthy and fit, their family histories of high cholesterol keep them on their toes. "Healthy cooking is a challenge I enjoy," she says.

Melani makes her livelihood as a freelance artist. Fittingly, one of her favorite types of assignments is painting food still lifes. And when she's not painting? Melani says that she enjoys bicycling and walking but finds that keeping up with her growing family gives her plenty of exercise. That's easy to understand, since the 35-year-old mom has a 3-year-old daughter and another child on the way.

Vibrant Rice and Chicken Soup

3 skinless chicken breast halves
4 cups water
1 can (14 ounces) low-sodium chicken stock
1 onion, chopped
3 carrots, sliced
2½ cups cooked Uncle Ben's Converted Rice
3 tablespoons lime juice
⅛ teaspoon ground cayenne pepper
1 small avocado, cubed
2 tomatoes, cubed
3 tablespoons minced fresh coriander
4 ounces queso fresco or farmer cheese, cubed

In a 4-quart pot over medium heat, bring the chicken, water, stock and onions to a boil. Reduce the heat and simmer for 25 minutes. Add the carrots and simmer for 20 minutes.

Remove the chicken from the pot and set aside until cool enough to handle. Remove the bones and cut the chicken into bite-size pieces.

Return the chicken to the pot. Stir in the rice, lime juice and pepper. Heat for 3 to 5 minutes, but don't boil.

Stir in the avocados, tomatoes and coriander. Heat through.

Divide the cheese among 4 soup bowls. Add the soup.

Serves 4

Per serving: 409 calories, 11.1 grams fat (24% of calories), 3.6 grams dietary fiber, 33.8 grams protein, 65 milligrams cholesterol, 125 milligrams sodium. Also a very good source of the B vitamins and vitamin A, vitamin C, calcium, iron and potassium. Also a good source of zinc.

SECOND PRIZE. Marjorie "GeGe" Kingston, Stockbridge, Massachusetts, for her Celebration Rice.

As its name suggests, this rice dish is a real celebration for your taste buds. It flavors crunchy roasted sesame seeds and wild rice with lively spices and a hint of citrus. "I love rice, and the contest stood for a lot of what I believe in," says GeGe. She was inspired by the contest's focus on healthy cooking to create this recipe.

In addition to cooking healthy meals, GeGe walks three miles daily to stay fit. This energetic hatmaker is definitely a woman on the go.

Celebration Rice

¾ cup Uncle Ben's Brown Rice
¼ cup wild rice
2 cups water
⅓ cup orange juice
1 tablespoon low-sodium soy sauce
1½ teaspoons olive oil
1 teaspoon grated orange rind
1 teaspoon curry powder
1 tablespoon toasted sesame seeds
2 tablespoons chopped chives or scallions
2 tablespoons chopped sweet red peppers

In a 2-quart saucepan over medium heat, stir the brown rice and wild rice until lightly toasted, about 5 minutes.

Add the water, orange juice, soy sauce, oil, orange rind and curry powder. Cover the pan tightly and cook over low heat for 45 to 50 minutes, or until all the liquid has been absorbed and the rice is tender.

Fluff the rice with a fork. Stir in the sesame seeds, chives or scallions and peppers.

Serves 4

Per serving: 119 calories, 3.4 grams fat (26% of calories), 0.8 gram dietary fiber, 3.6 grams protein, no cholesterol, 156 milligrams sodium. Also a very good source of vitamin A, vitamin C, thiamine, niacin and folacin. Also a good source of zinc.

THIRD PRIZE. Virginia Moon, Harvest, Alabama, for her Herbed Rice Bread.

Low in fat and flavored with mixed herbs and a dusting of Parmesan cheese, this unique rice-and-cornmeal bread is a real delight.

Virginia came up with the bread recipe while looking for a new use for rice, a food commonly found on her family's dinner table. "I'm a lacto-ovo [milk and egg] vegetarian, but because I love foods like rice, I don't feel I sacrifice a thing to maintain this type of diet," says Virginia.

The 32-year-old cook keeps her shape by walking, jogging and cycling. She makes it a point to fit exercise into her daily routine.

Herbed Rice Bread
1 cup white cornmeal
1 tablespoon grated Parmesan cheese
1 teaspoon baking powder
1 teaspoon onion powder
½ teaspoon garlic powder
½ teaspoon dried mixed herbs, such as fines herbes
¼ teaspoon salt (optional)
¼ cup fat-free egg substitute or 2 egg whites
1 cup skim milk
¼ cup nonfat sour cream or yogurt
1 cup cold cooked Uncle Ben's Converted Rice
1 tablespoon light margarine, melted

In a small bowl, mix the cornmeal, Parmesan, baking powder, onion powder, garlic powder, herbs and salt.

In a large bowl, whisk the egg substitute or egg whites until frothy. Whisk in the milk and sour cream or yogurt. Stir in the dry ingredients.

Place the rice in a small bowl. Drizzle with margarine. Mix and mash the rice with a fork or potato masher. Add to the cornmeal mixture and stir to combine.

Coat an 8" baking dish with no-stick spray. Add the batter. Bake at 400° for 30 minutes.

Serves 9

Per serving: 113 calories, 1.2 grams fat (10% of calories), 1 gram dietary fiber, 4.2 grams protein, 1 milligram cholesterol, 92 milligrams sodium. Also a very good source of vitamin A, thiamine, folacin, vitamin B_6, vitamin B_{12} and calcium.

Vegetarian Entrées

FIRST PRIZE. Martha Jane Parasida, Baden, Pennsylvania, for her Polenta, Bean and Pasta Casserole.

Sautéed peppers and onions give this all-in-one meal its zing, but that's not the only pleasant surprise. An assortment of beans and cornmeal creates a fiber-rich meal that's low in fat and sodium. "I see nutrition and fitness as going hand in hand," explains Martha Jane. She and her husband began exercising regularly about 15 years ago. That's about the same time they discovered the benefits of cooking for health, too. The results of their commitment are immeasurable. "Our weight has stayed down so easily that we don't even worry about it," she says.

"I love the challenge of making old recipes healthier," says Martha Jane, a 45-year-old hairdresser who notes that her conversations with clients at the salon provide the inspiration and ideas for her best recipe makeovers.

Polenta, Bean and Pasta Casserole

½ cup cornmeal
½ cup cold water
1½ cups boiling water
½ cup corn
¼ cup wheat germ
1 green pepper, chopped
4 scallions, chopped
1 teaspoon olive oil
¼ teaspoon herbal salt substitute
2 ounces brick cheese, shredded
4 ounces uncooked penne or mostaccioli pasta
2 cups cooked black-eyed peas or kidney beans
1½ cups salsa or tomato sauce

In a 2-quart saucepan, stir together the cornmeal and cold water. Slowly whisk in the boiling water. Bring to a boil over medium heat and cook, stirring constantly, for 10 minutes, or until thick. Stir in the corn and wheat germ. Set aside.

Coat a 10" × 10" casserole dish or 9" × 13" baking dish with no-stick spray. Spread the cornmeal mixture

93

evenly over the bottom of the dish. Refrigerate while preparing the topping.

In a large no-stick frying pan, stir-fry the green peppers and scallions in the oil. Sprinkle with the salt substitute. Spread over the cornmeal mixture. Sprinkle with the cheese. Set aside.

Cook the pasta in a large pot of boiling water until just tender, about 7 minutes. Drain and place in a large bowl. Add the peas or beans and salsa or tomato sauce. Mix well and pour over the vegetables and cornmeal mixture in the casserole dish.

Cover with a lid. Microwave on high (100% power) for a total of 10 to 12 minutes, rotating the dish a quarter turn 3 times during this period; let stand for 5 minutes. (Or bake at 350° for about 20 minutes.)

Cut into squares. If desired, serve with extra salsa or sauce.

Serves 4

Per serving: 382 calories, 9.5 grams fat (22% of calories), 9.4 grams dietary fiber, 14.4 grams protein, 13 milligrams cholesterol, 427 milligrams sodium. Also a very good source of the B vitamins, vitamin C, vitamin A, calcium, zinc, potassium and iron.

SECOND PRIZE. Linda Vibbert, Glasgow, Kentucky, for her Vegetarian Chili.

With all the hot and spicy taste of traditional chili, this nutritious meal uses bulgur in place of ground beef. It's a creative way to make an old favorite into a new vegetarian treat.

Linda says that she gets a good feeling knowing she is preparing healthy foods for herself and others. She's been doing so for about three years, along with walking regularly.

"I go walking during breaks or over lunch," she says. This activity, and better eating habits, has definitely helped Linda look and feel great.

Vegetarian Chili

2 cups tomato juice
½ cup bulgur
1 onion, chopped
1 carrot, chopped
½ green pepper, chopped
2 tablespoons olive oil
1½ tablespoons chili powder
1 teaspoon ground cumin
½ teaspoon dried oregano
¼ teaspoon garlic powder
¼ teaspoon ground red pepper
¼ teaspoon ground black pepper
1 teaspoon honey
1 can (about 14 ounces) tomatoes, coarsely chopped
2 cups cooked kidney beans
2 ounces mild canned green chili peppers, chopped

In a 1-quart saucepan over medium heat, bring the tomato juice to a boil. Stir in the bulgur. Cover, remove from heat, and set aside.

In a 3-quart saucepan over medium heat, sauté the onions, carrots and green peppers in the oil until tender, about 5 minutes. Add the chili powder, cumin, oregano, garlic powder, red pepper, black pepper and honey. Stir for 1 minute. Stir in the tomatoes (with their juice), beans and chili peppers.

Fluff the bulgur mixture with a fork. Add to the pan. Bring to a boil, then reduce the heat and simmer for 20 minutes.

Serves 4

Per serving: 319 calories, 8.9 grams fat (25% of calories), 14.5 grams dietary fiber, 12.8 grams protein, no cholesterol, 537 milligrams sodium. Also a very good source of vitamin A, the B vitamins, vitamin C, iron, zinc, calcium and potassium.

THIRD PRIZE. Margaret Donohue, Bellevue, Nebraska, for her Hearty Eggplant-Barley Bake.
Since Margaret coaches endurance athletes and runs

marathons, you can be sure her eggplant dish is premium fuel that's low in fat. Plus, it tastes terrific! Margaret makes sure she eats light and avoids meats most of the time. As a distance runner, she knows from experience the importance of good nutrition.

Hearty Eggplant-Barley Bake

½ cup chopped onions
½ cup chopped mushrooms
¼ cup chopped green peppers
1 tablespoon minced garlic
1 teaspoon olive oil
1 cup cubed eggplant
2 tablespoons water
1 can (16 ounces) tomatoes, chopped
1½ cups water
¾ cup quick-cooking barley
½ cup chili sauce
¼ cup chopped fresh parsley
1 teaspoon honey
1 teaspoon Worcestershire sauce
½ teaspoon dried marjoram
¼ teaspoon ground black pepper

In a large no-stick frying pan over medium heat, sauté the onions, mushrooms, green peppers and garlic in the oil until softened, about 5 minutes. Add the eggplant and 2 tablespoons water; sauté until softened, about 10 minutes.

Add the tomatoes (with their juice), 1½ cups water, barley, chili sauce, parsley, honey, Worcestershire sauce, marjoram and black pepper. Bring to a boil, then reduce heat and simmer for 20 minutes, or until the barley is tender.

Serves 4

Per serving: 224 calories, 2 grams fat (8% of calories), 7.3 grams dietary fiber, 6.5 grams protein, no cholesterol, 439 milligrams sodium. Also a very good source of vitamin A, the B vitamins, vitamin C, iron and potassium. Also a good source of calcium.

Fish and Seafood

FIRST PRIZE. Elizabeth Goldstein, Yardley, Pennsylvania, for her Tuna Curry Sandwich.

A most unlikely combination—curry, mustard, tuna and, yes, banana—made a winner out of this sandwich. This exotic concoction gives a tangy, pungent twist to everyday tuna.

Elizabeth's family teased her about entering "that crazy sandwich" into a recipe contest. The last laugh was Elizabeth's, however. The curry and tuna delight turned out to be not only unusual and delicious but quite healthy, too.

The 22-year-old law school student became health conscious after realizing that poor eating habits and a sedentary lifestyle had made it difficult for her to relax and concentrate on her studies. Now, she makes an effort to keep her meals nutritious and to exercise on her stationary bike as often as she can.

Tuna Curry Sandwich

1 can (6½ ounces) water-packed albacore tuna,
    drained and flaked
¼ cup chopped onions
2 tablespoons low-fat mayonnaise
1 teaspoon Dijon mustard
½ teaspoon curry powder
1 banana, sliced
4 slices pumpernickel or rye bread
4 cucumber slices (optional)

In a medium bowl, combine the tuna, onions, mayonnaise, mustard and curry powder. Fold in the bananas.

Spread the mixture on 2 slices of the bread. Top with the cucumbers and remaining bread.

Serves 2

Per serving: 369 calories, 8.4 grams fat (20% of calories), 5 grams dietary fiber, 26.9 grams protein, 37 milligrams cholesterol, 676 milligrams sodium. Also a good source of niacin, vitamin B_6, vitamin B_{12}, iron, potassium and omega-3's.

SECOND PRIZE. Alex Fotopoulos, Cresskill, New Jersey, for his Grecian Scallop Salad.

The dressing on this seafood salad packs a spicy tomato-and-vinaigrette punch that is bound to please. Try this unique variation of seafood salad as your next cold meal.

Alex, who loves seafood, created this dish to meet more than just his high standards of taste. "I started cooking low-fat recipes when I finished law school and noticed I needed to shed a few pounds," says Alex. We are pleased to report that he has lost 45 pounds since he started eating low-fat foods and working out, just over a year ago.

Grecian Scallop Salad

Salad

16 medium sea scallops
2 tablespoons lemon juice
1 teaspoon water
½ tablespoon garlic powder
3 cups chopped romaine lettuce
2 medium tomatoes, chopped
1 medium cucumber, chopped
1 cup cooked rice
2 tablespoons crumbled feta cheese

Vinaigrette

¼ cup red wine vinegar
1½ tablespoons balsamic vinegar
1 tablespoon olive oil
1½ tablespoons minced fresh parsley
1 tablespoon dried basil
1 teaspoon garlic powder
1 teaspoon hot-pepper sauce (optional)
¼ teaspoon dried oregano
⅛ teaspoon ground black pepper
1 cup crushed tomatoes
¼ cup diced onions

To make the salad: Coat a large no-stick frying pan with no-stick spray. Over medium heat, sauté the scallops for a few minutes. Add the lemon juice, water and garlic powder. Cook another few minutes, until the scallops are cooked. Set aside to cool.

In a large bowl, toss together the lettuce, tomatoes and cucumbers. Cover with the rice, then the scallops. Sprinkle with the feta. Set aside.

To make the vinaigrette: In a large bowl, whisk together the red wine vinegar, balsamic vinegar, oil, parsley, basil, garlic powder, hot-pepper sauce, oregano and pepper. Mix in the tomatoes and onions.

Pour over the salad and toss well.

Serves 4

Per serving: 208 calories, 6 grams fat (26% of calories), 3.9 grams dietary fiber, 11.9 grams protein, 19 milligrams cholesterol, 162 milligrams sodium. Also a very good source of vitamin A, the B vitamins, vitamin C, calcium, iron, zinc and potassium.

THIRD PRIZE. Randolph Bush, Trumbull, Connecticut, for his Ginger Snapper.

This ginger-sautéed red snapper deserves an award not only for great taste but for super nutrition as well. The spicy sauce and distinctive snapper flavor aren't the only perks to this dish. The entrée is also high in protein and a good source of vitamins B_6 and B_{12}, and only 23 percent of its calories come from fat.

Randy has always enjoyed cooking and uses the hobby as a way to relieve stress. This contest was his first. (And it's doubtful it will be the last!)

Ginger Snapper

Sauce
1 scallion, thinly sliced
2 tablespoons minced shallots
1 tablespoon freshly grated ginger
½ teaspoon olive oil
1 cup defatted chicken stock
1 ounce flaked crab (optional)

Snapper
4 red snapper fillets (4 ounces each)
1 tablespoon powdered ginger
¼ cup cornstarch
2 teaspoons olive oil

99

To make the sauce: In a 1-quart saucepan over medium heat, sauté the scallions, shallots and ginger in the oil for 3 minutes. Add the stock. Raise the heat to high and boil until the stock is reduced by half.

Reduce the heat to low and stir in the crab. Keep warm.

To make the snapper: Sprinkle the snapper with the ginger. Place the cornstarch in a small sieve and shake over the fish to coat on all sides.

In a large no-stick frying pan over medium-high heat, heat the oil. Add the fish and sauté for about 4 minutes per side. Transfer the fish to serving plates and spoon the sauce over it.

Serves 4

Per serving: 187 calories, 4.8 grams fat (23% of calories), 23.8 grams protein, 42 milligrams cholesterol, 94 milligrams sodium. Also a very good source of vitamin B_6 and vitamin B_{12}.

Desserts

FIRST PRIZE. Ellen Burr, Truro, Massachusetts, for her Oriental Aromatica Rice Pudding.

Oriental five-spice powder and grated tangerine rind are the secret ingredients that make this rice pudding unforgettable.

It's a low-fat dessert guaranteed to become a favorite your family will ask for again and again.

"I'm so glad this recipe won. It's an old family favorite," says Ellen, who is also a Cape Cod forager (someone who collects food from the environment). She plans to pass on her healthy cooking and living traditions to her daughter so that generations to follow will reap the benefits she has gained. "I feel like now I have considerably more energy to do the things I like to do. I gave up smoking about five years ago and try to maintain a healthy lifestyle these days. I find it's definitely paid off," says Ellen.

Oriental Aromatica Rice Pudding

1 cup aromatic rice
1 tablespoon canola oil
1 tablespoon grated tangerine or orange rind
1 teaspoon five-spice powder
2 cups water
1 can (15 ounces) evaporated skim milk
½ cup chopped dates
¼ cup chopped dried black figs
2 tablespoons minced crystallized ginger
2 tablespoons toasted pine nuts
   ground cinnamon

In a 3-quart saucepan over medium heat, stir the rice and oil until glossy, about 5 minutes. Stir in the tangerine or orange rind and five-spice powder. Add the water. Boil, reduce heat, cover; simmer for 20 minutes.

Stir in the milk, dates and figs. Cook over low heat, stirring often, until the mixture is thick and creamy.

Serve warm, sprinkled with the ginger, pine nuts and cinnamon.

Serves 6

Per serving: 272 calories, 4.5 grams fat (15% of calories), 2.4 grams dietary fiber, 9 grams protein, 3 milligrams cholesterol, 87 milligrams sodium. Also a very good source of vitamin A, the B vitamins, calcium, iron, zinc and potassium.

SECOND PRIZE. Gloria Bradley, Naperville, Illinois, for her Pear-Raspberry Clafouti.

Gloria recommends trying this goody in place of ice cream. It's a low-fat, high-fiber dessert that will delight any sweet tooth.

Gloria is a retired database specialist who loves to cook. Her philosophy is that healthy meals are more scrumptious than regular ones because they require fresh foods and creative ideas.

In addition to being a great cook, she makes time every week to play golf, practice her tennis and work out. "By staying active and eating right, I not only feel better, I look better, too," says Gloria.

Pear-Raspberry Clafouti

1 can (29 ounces) pear halves, drained and chopped
¾ cup rolled oats
1 cup skim milk
½ cup fat-free egg substitute
2 tablespoons vanilla
1 tablespoon honey
1 teaspoon grated lemon rind
½ cup raspberries
¼ teaspoon ground cinnamon
nonfat frozen raspberry yogurt (optional)

Coat a deep 9" pie plate with no-stick spray. Spread the pears in an even layer in the dish.

Place the oats in a blender. Cover and process on high for 1 minute, or until finely chopped. Add the milk, egg substitute, vanilla, honey and lemon rind. Process until well blended, stopping occasionally to scrape down the sides of the blender.

Gently ladle the batter over the pears. Sprinkle with the raspberries and cinnamon. Bake at 350° for 35 to 40 minutes, or until puffed and cooked through. Cool slightly. Serve plain or with the frozen yogurt.

Serves 6

Per serving: 113 calories, 0.8 gram fat (6% of calories), 2.3 grams dietary fiber, 4.9 grams protein, no cholesterol, 50 milligrams sodium. A source of vitamin C, thiamine, vitamin B_{12}, calcium and potassium.

THIRD PRIZE. Angela Bond, Wilkesboro, North Carolina, for her Good-for-You Fruity Cake.

Fresh fruits and honey-spiced syrup make this a treat truly rich in flavor, but it's much lower in fat than traditional fruitcakes.

Angela first became interested in healthy cooking to lower her family's high cholesterol. The results have been inspiring.

"My husband and I both had cholesterol levels exceeding 200. Mine is now down to about 150, and his is down to about 170. We attribute our success to a better diet and taking a three-mile walk every day," she says.

Good-for-You Fruity Cake

Cake
⅔ cup whole-wheat flour
⅔ cup unbleached flour
½ cup quick-cooking rolled oats
1½ teaspoons baking soda
1 teaspoon ground cinnamon
4 egg whites
⅓ cup honey
¼ cup canola oil
1 teaspoon vanilla
⅓ cup orange juice
¾ cup shredded apples or pears
½ cup cranberries
¼ cup raisins
¼ cup chopped dates

Orange Syrup
½ cup orange juice
⅓ cup honey
½ teaspoon ground cinnamon

To make the cake: In a large bowl, combine the whole-wheat flour, unbleached flour, oats, baking soda and cinnamon.

In a medium bowl, whisk together the egg whites and honey. Whisk in the oil and vanilla, then the orange juice. Stir in the apples or pears, cranberries, raisins and dates.

Pour the fruit mixture over the dry ingredients. Fold until the dry ingredients are just moistened; do not overmix.

Coat a 9" × 13" baking dish with no-stick spray. Add the batter and spread evenly. Bake at 350° for 20 to 25 minutes, or until browned and firm to the touch. Remove from the oven and place on a wire rack.

To make the syrup: In a 1-quart saucepan over medium heat, cook together the orange juice, honey and cinnamon until syrupy. Pour over the hot cake. Serve warm or cold.

Serves 10

Per serving: 235 calories, 6 grams fat (23% of calories), 2.2 grams dietary fiber, 4.1 grams protein, no cholesterol, 148 milligrams sodium. Also a very good source of the B vitamins, vitamin C, iron and potassium.

103

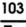

9 "Desalt" Your Blood Pressure Problems

People who exercise, lose weight and shake sodium from their diets can cut blood pressure down to size.

By George Blackburn, M.D., Ph.D.

What's a Caesar salad without anchovies? A Chinese dinner without soy sauce? Mom's chicken soup without salt?

Nothing, if not for the blood pressure benefits bestowed on those of us who abstain from the S-word.

Sodium—as in sodium chloride (table salt), sodium bicarbonate (baking soda) and sodium citrate (a preservative)—has long been blacklisted from a heart-healthy diet. That's because sodium may contribute to high blood pressure (a major cause of heart attack, stroke and kidney disease). We're not exactly sure how.

We do know that regularly consuming excessive amounts of salt, which is about 40 percent sodium, can bring on high blood pressure in some people. In fact, a study of more than 10,000 people in 32 countries showed a direct correlation between dietary salt and elevation of blood pressure: The higher the salt intake, the higher the blood pressure. That's bad news. But it's worth noting that about 50 percent of the people with high blood pressure are sodium-sensitive. For the majority of the population, eating salty foods does not appear to bring on or exacerbate blood pressure problems as do overeating and being overweight.

Beyond Sodium

If you have high blood pressure, you need to discuss your diet with your physician, since many people with high blood pressure are salt-sensitive. But, in general, the best approach to prevent and control moderately high

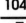

blood pressure is one that involves multiple lifestyle factors, including a healthy diet, weight control and exercise.

In a recent study, about 100 men and women with "high-normal" blood pressure were encouraged to lower their sodium intake to under 1,800 milligrams (less than the amount in one teaspoon of salt) as well as to lose some weight, cut back on alcohol and exercise moderately. Although only 13 percent of participants met the sodium goal, their incidence of hypertension at the end of five years was less than half that of a similar group who did not go through all the changes.

Most of the people in the study group exercised more, lost an average of 4½ pounds and reported drinking 30 percent less alcohol.

This doesn't mean we can bring back the saltshaker. As I mentioned, most of the excess sodium comes from the saltshaker. Moreover, overindulging in salty food causes water retention and taxes the kidneys. Plus, there's preliminary evidence that a high-salt diet may damage blood vessels regardless of blood pressure.

Besides, we're simply eating far too much of the stuff.

It's true that the body requires a small amount of sodium to help nerves and muscles function properly—and, believe it or not, to keep blood volume and pressure normal. We're talking about a tiny amount, less than ¼ teaspoon of salt each day, which should be easily provided by a good diet.

The typical American has developed a salt craving, consuming twice the safe and adequate amount a day (according to the National Research Council). That's why experts say it's wise to keep a lid on salt intake. Challenge yourself to make a 25 percent reduction in your daily salt intake. But do not lose sight of other lifestyle factors that can help you meet your blood pressure goals.

Cut the Sodium with the Fat

Many of my patients with high blood pressure tell me that they don't use salt at all. But they're still overweight. My guess is that because many of them focus so much on totally excluding sodium, their foods are bland.

105
■

So what happens? They're heavy-handed with fats like butter, oil and margarine to make food taste better.

Think for a minute about your diet priorities. You know that enemy number one is fat. In fact, lowering the fat in your diet is of utmost importance in controlling your cholesterol and your weight. As it turns out, many of the high-fat foods you should avoid eating—like salami, hot dogs, potato chips and cheeses—are also high in salt. So cutting them out will do your heart good on two counts.

Not surprisingly, too, the foods you should eat in order to follow a low-fat diet are naturally low in sodium: unprocessed grains, fruits (fresh, frozen and canned), vegetables (fresh and frozen without salt), low-fat milk and yogurt, and fresh lean meats, poultry and fish. By eating this way, you'll also be getting calcium and potassium, which also play a role in maintaining healthy blood pressure.

The reality is that if overweight people followed low-fat diets, they'd be likely to permanently lose some weight (a five-pound drop can substantially lower blood pressure) and at the same time find that their diet is automatically lower in sodium.

More Sodium-Trimming Tips

Of course, if you focus on lean and naturally low-sodium foods but douse them with table salt or salty condiments, you're defeating the purpose. Here are a few other tips to help you moderate a salty palate.

■ When preparing foods, spice them up with naturally low-sodium flavorings: lemon and lime juice, herbs and spices, and herb vinegars. Make your own salt-free herb blends with combinations like garlic powder, basil and oregano. Use chopped onion and garlic liberally.

■ Read food labels. Choose low-sodium or reduced-sodium products whenever possible. To make the claim "reduced sodium" on a label, a product must have at least 75 percent less sodium than the usual version of the food. A "low-sodium" food must have no more than 140 milligrams of sodium per serving. "Very low sodium" means 35 milligrams or less per serving.

■ Use salty condiments sparingly. One anchovy fillet divided four ways in a Caesar salad can add a surprising amount of flavor for just 36 milligrams of sodium per serving. Just remember, if you use sodium-containing condiments, skip any added table salt.

■ Save your saltshaker for those foods that positively won't make it without a pinch, like chicken soup, gazpacho or homemade bread. (Salt is needed in yeast breads to control the action of yeast, but the amounts of salt are usually small.)

■ Under no circumstances salt the water when boiling pasta or cooking rice. There's absolutely no need for it. And believe me, you won't know the difference.

■ Omit salt from recipes or cut the amount of salt in half, whenever possible.

One final note about sodium: Studies show that people who gradually reduce the amount they use eventually lose their desire for salty foods. Allow five weeks to desalt your taste buds.

10   Nutritional Power Plans

America's top nutritionists compile their "A" lists.

Of all the hundreds of dietary habits you can possibly adopt, which ones are the most powerful for preventing disease and promoting optimum health? Should you put a lot of energy into reducing the amount of cholesterol in your diet? The amount of sodium?

Or is it more important to avoid irradiated food or alcoholic beverages? In other words, where exactly is the biggest health payoff? This question was posed to over 300 top nutrition experts. These black belts in nutrition were asked to rate 44 nutritional actions (all purported to benefit health) as follows: extremely important, very important, important, not important, but may help or probably worthless.

The nutritionists' responses were then compiled and statistically weighted to create a list of dietary "top priorities" for preserving and boosting your health.

"We could easily have an enormous advance in the health of America if we could simply follow the priorities of the nation's knowledgeable nutritionists," says George L. Blackburn, M.D., Ph.D., associate professor at Harvard Medical School.

Setting Priorities

So here's what the experts say about what's really vital in your diet, what's not so crucial and what's not worth worrying about.

Get the Fat Out ▶ Although the experts polled came from widely diverse areas of nutrition research—from cancer to heart disease, from food science to geriatrics—they delivered their message about the number-one diet priority like a choir in perfect harmony: If you do anything, control your weight! Ninety-seven percent of the experts polled gave weight control high priority.

"Overweight is a big problem in the United States," says Kelly Brownell, Ph.D., professor of psychology at Yale University and a top obesity researcher.

"It's affecting more and more people. It's creeping down lower into the age brackets, so there are more and more overweight youngsters." According to a nationwide survey of America's health behavior conducted by Louis Harris and Associates, nearly two-thirds of U.S. adults are overweight for their age, build and sex. And fewer than half of them say they tried to lose weight in the past month.

That's a tragedy, because obesity not only is an independent risk factor for increased mortality but also contributes to diseases such as heart disease, high blood pressure, diabetes and gallbladder disease. "If everybody in the United States maintained their ideal weight, the incidence of Type II diabetes would be greatly reduced, hypertension would be much less common, and so would coronary disease," says Meir Stampfer, M.D., Dr.P.H., associate professor of epidemiology at Harvard School of Public Health. Obesity is clearly one of the biggest challenges we face in health today.

The number of calories you eat is the ultimate determinant of how much you will weigh. But because cutting calories almost always involves cutting fat, both these actions scored very high with experts. Seventy-five percent said that cutting calories was extremely important or very important; 70 percent said the same about controlling fat intake. And of course, cutting dietary fat is good for other reasons: It helps slash the risk of heart disease by halting or even reversing the plaque buildup that chokes arteries, and it may cut the risk of some forms of cancer.

Those two themes, controlling weight and controlling fat intake, seem to cut across the whole spectrum of diseases that ravage Americans as we age.

Rev Up Your Engine ▶ The next order of business, according to the nutrition pros: Put your body in motion. Eighty-four percent of them gave high priority to increasing your physical activity to enable greater nutrient intake.

These top-flight nutritionists know that there's more than one route to rotundity. People pile on the pounds when they eat too much and when they exercise too little. By the same token, "it's hard to reduce your weight by controlling calories alone," says Dr. Stampfer. "If you exercise as well, you're more likely to be able to maintain the weight loss in the long run."

What's more, by burning calories, exercise allows you to eat more. That's important because it's hard to get enough nutrients when dieting. In fact, it's hard even if you're not dieting.

"U.S. Department of Agriculture surveys show that the average American woman eats less than 1,800 calories a day," says Judith S. Stern, R.D., Sc.D., a professor of nutrition at the University of California, Davis. "It's difficult to meet the Recommended Dietary Allowances (RDAs) for vitamins and minerals on that amount of food, unless your choices are extremely lean and nutrient dense."

Exercise also helps lower blood pressure, relieve stress and keep your ticker and circulatory system in top form. And it helps your bones stay brawny. "You can eat all the calcium in the world," says Dr. Blackburn, "and if you don't exercise your body, you're not going to have strong bones." Most people can fill their exercise quota with just 20 minutes of brisk walking three times a week.

Enjoy Your Food ▶ The nutritionists also ranked as a top priority something that too many diet schemes leave out: enjoying your food. Eighty-seven percent of the nutritionists thought that food enjoyment was important. At first look, that doesn't seem to square with their emphasis on weight loss. "One problem with the American diet is that people enjoy the food too much," says Dr. Brownell. "The fact that there are widely available high-calorie, high-fat foods that taste good is part of the problem. But having nutritious foods that taste better certainly would be a priority."

In other words, nobody is going to eat food they don't enjoy. If you want to eat healthy, you're going to have to learn how to cook low-fat dishes that taste great.

Make Your Meals a Medley ▶ It used to be the nutritionist's creed: Balance your diet among the four food groups and make sure you get the RDA for vitamins and minerals. And these concepts are certainly not passé— roughly 90 percent of those surveyed said they're still high priority. Yet those concepts now clearly take a backseat to cutting fat and controlling weight.

It seems that the weakness of the four-food-groups approach is that it doesn't provide enough guidance to prevent you from gobbling up too much fat and amassing too much fat on your body.

If you make fat fighting your number-one priority, however, it quite naturally leads you toward fulfilling those other guidelines. "If you phase out the high-calorie, high-fat foods in your diet, you're going to have to replace them with something low-fat—cereals, fruits and vegetables," says Dr. Blackburn, who is also chief of the Nutrition/Metabolism Laboratory at New England Deaconess Hospital, Boston. An emphasis on those foods moves you closer to meeting your RDA for vitamins and minerals. It can also move you closer to balancing your diet, which for most Americans is overladen with high-fat meat and dairy products.

Set Your Fat Priorities ▶ Trading in saturated fats for heart-smarter monounsaturated and polyunsaturated fats has been the talk of the town lately. But the nutritionists clearly consider this to be fine-tuning, not top priority. "You can't put the cart before the horse," says Dr. Blackburn. "It's far more important to cut the total amount of fat in your diet."

The nutritionists recommend the American Heart Association's cutoff—30 percent of calories from fat—as the upper limit. (Many doctors recommend aiming even lower.) "Once you've done that, you can try to take another bite out of saturated fat," says Dr. Blackburn.

Rest assured, though, that even in meeting the 30 percent limit you will be cutting most of your saturated fat intake. That's because most of the all-American foods that are highest in total fat—ice cream, cheeseburgers, doughnuts, for example—are the very same foods that are highest in saturated fat.

Weeding out the cholesterol in your diet is considered less useful than banishing saturated fat. Only 14 percent of the nutritionists rated this "extremely important." That's because the excess saturated fat you eat raises your blood cholesterol more than the extra cholesterol you eat. Also, foods can have no cholesterol yet still be dangerously high in fat.

Quest for Fiber ▶ The country's top nutrition experts were solidly behind boosting fiber intake to at least 20 grams per day. The specific type of fiber—soluble or insoluble—is less important, they say. "We eat so little fiber, we'll take anything," says Dr. Blackburn. "Whatever you can find—some peas in your stew—put it in!"

A high-fiber diet fills you up without filling you out, keeps you regular, helps lower your cholesterol level and may help reduce the risk of colon cancer. Fruits, vegetables, whole grains and legumes top the fiber charts.

Don't Fear to Say Cheers—Occasionally ▶ The nation's top nutritionists plainly don't support prohibiting alcoholic beverages. But they're staunch believers in moderation. "There's no evidence, unless you are pregnant or driving, that drinking alcohol in limited quantities is bad for you," says Dr. Stern. Alcohol in excess can become "demon rum." Then it destroys livers as well as lives.

Practice Safe Eating ▶ While many people are worried about pesticides on fruit and vegetables, the experts rated it 34 out of 44 on their list of priorities. But more than three-quarters of the nutritionists thought it wise to avoid certain raw foods—eggs, meat and seafood. Raw eggs and chicken can house salmonella bacteria, a common cause of food poisoning. Raw seafood can harbor viruses or parasites. Buy only from a reputable dealer or avoid raw seafood altogether.

Eat More Surf, Less Turf ▶ The experts also placed a high priority on replacing meat with fish and cutting meat portions to three to four ounces. Both help shave down fat, especially saturated. If you're an inveterate meat lover or a fishaphobic, however, there's still hope. Look to lean cuts, such as flank steak, and to low-fat cooking methods, such as broiling and braising.

Be Wary of "Scares" ▶ The nutritionists in general were not supportive of nutrition scares. Avoiding trans-fatty acids (found in stick margarine), tropical oils and sugar drew only moderate priority ratings from the nutrition authorities. You may find that surprising, considering the bad press those three have gotten. But trans-fatty acids (similar to saturated fats) and tropical oils (rich in saturated fat of vegetable origin) actually make up only a small percentage of our diet, and they have not been proven harmful. Again, better to concentrate on reducing all types of fat than to focus on this micro-issue. Sugar is a problem for people who are obese (it packs lots of calories without much nutritional clout) or diabetic (they can't metabolize it properly). For the rest of us, though, the pros feel avoiding sugar is not of utmost importance.

Have It Your Way ▶ The experts gave only a moderate priority rating to avoiding snacks and eating three square meals a day. It seems the nutrition masters are trying to tell us something: What you eat is much more important than how you eat.

Medical
Care
Updates

Give the Slip to Cystitis

Tips for preventing—and treating—this uncomfortable urinary complaint.

When Lisa Jacobson was in graduate school, she picked up more than an education. It was also her first introduction to cystitis—a urinary tract infection (UTI). The symptoms came on fast and furiously, she says, with fierce pain and stinging every time she urinated. And always there was that uncomfortable feeling that she needed to go again, even if she had just done so minutes before.

Her doctor identified the culprit—bacteria in her bladder—and immediately prescribed an antibiotic. She recovered quickly and thought that was the end of it. But soon the symptoms returned, and she needed to be treated again. The problem persisted, on and off, for more than two years, until finally a urologist put her on a longer course of antibiotic treatment, which seemed to do the trick. Or so she thought.

A few years later, however, Lisa's bladder symptoms erupted once more. But unlike her bouts in the past, this attack could not be traced to bladder bacteria. And so, Lisa's search for a solution began all over again.

A Common Complaint

Lisa's experience, unfortunately, is not unique. Cystitis, usually caused by a bacterial infection, is second only to colds in prevalence in women, says Kristene Whitmore, M.D., clinical associate professor of urology at the University of Pennsylvania and chief of urology at Graduate Hospital in Philadelphia. And while it's usually an easy-to-diagnose, easy-to-treat condition, for 15 percent of those afflicted, bladder infections persist, recurring often and with frustrating regularity—sometimes only weeks or months apart. Occasionally, too, a bacterium does not appear to be the only trigger.

Doctors admit that there's a lot they do not understand about this problem. But, they say, promising theories are yielding new treatments with positive results.

The Bacterial Connection

Women are prime targets because the female anatomy makes it more convenient for *Escherichia coli* bacteria, which normally inhabit the colon, to travel from the rectum to the vagina, up the urethra and into the bladder. *E. coli* infections are considered the primary culprit in cystitis.

It's important to understand that in most women bacteria enter the bladder without causing an infection. The germs are simply flushed out with the urine, says Dr. Whitmore.

Sometimes there's a breakdown in the bladder's natural defenses. Concentration of urine and pooling of urine in the bladder can increase the risk that errant bacteria will multiply and cause a bladder infection.

If cystitis takes hold, there's no mistaking it. With the subtlety of a steamroller, the symptoms appear: burning and pain on urination, an urgency to urinate frequently, blood in the urine and, sometimes, a soreness in the lower abdomen or back.

Even if the symptoms could be ignored (which is extremely unlikely), it wouldn't be wise to do so. Left untreated, a bacterial infection can travel from the bladder to the kidneys, where it can inflict serious damage. See your doctor at the first sign of trouble.

A simple urinalysis can confirm suspicions. Since urine is normally sterile, the presence of bacteria is a good indication of infection. In addition to a standard urinalysis, your doctor may order a urine culture and sensitivity test. The culture tells your doctor exactly which bacteria are growing in the urine. (Usually it's a strain of *E. coli,* although other bacteria, such as staphylococcus and streptococcus, have been identified.) The sensitivity test helps determine which antibiotic the offending germs are most susceptible to.

The New Quick Cure

It used to be that a confirmed UTI was routinely treated with a 10- to 14-day course of antibiotics. This usually wiped out the infection, but at a cost. Excessive antibiotic treatment zaps good bacteria with bad. With a shortage of good bacteria (which normally keep the body's bad organisms in check and balance), you're vulnerable to other infections. For many women the trade-off is a vaginal yeast infection.

Today, doctors are adopting a more prudent approach.

"For as many as 80 to 90 percent of those with urinary tract infections, a single dose—just one to four pills at once—can wipe out the infection and the symptoms, especially for first-time or sporadic cases," says Dr. Whitmore. "Most doctors, though, give a three- to five-day course of treatment to be on the safe side. That's still far less than we used to prescribe, and so the likelihood of complications is greatly reduced."

Troublesome Cases

Fortunately, for most women, the quick cure ends cystitis forever. But for others, it's just a reprieve.

When bladder problems recur again and again—and repeated antibiotic treatment fails to put an end to them—doctors need to search further for the underlying cause. Additional diagnostic tests may be performed to rule out diabetes, kidney stones and other urinary tract disorders.

A new theory suggests that some of those susceptible to recurrent infections may have bladder walls that allow bacteria to "stick," making it more difficult for urination to wash them out, says Grant Mulholland, M.D., chairman of the Department of Urology at Thomas Jefferson University Hospital in Philadelphia.

In most cases, however, there is no one simple explanation. But there are many potential contributing factors, including the following.

Sexual Intercourse ▸ "During intercourse, bacteria from the surrounding areas can be pushed into the ure-

117

BLADDER-SAFE SEX

For many women, sex and cystitis go together like love and marriage. Consequently they may abstain out of fear of reinfection. Clearly, not a prescription for a happy relationship! Here are some better ideas.

• Urinate before and after sex. Drink water before sex so you'll have something to void afterward. This helps flush out any bacteria that may have entered.

• Use a hand-held shower after sex to wash germs from your vaginal area.

• If you use a diaphragm in combination with a spermicide, consider switching to another form of contraception for a while to see if it makes a difference. Or, at the very least, be sure your diaphragm is fitted properly so the rim doesn't obstruct the urethra.

thra by the back-and-forth motion of the penis," says Dr. Mulholland. "Some women get an infection almost every time they have sex."

Certain Contraceptives ▶ Studies have shown that women who use a diaphragm are two to four times more prone to recurrent infection than nonusers, says Dr. Whitmore. "The spring rim of the diaphragm can compress the bladder neck, causing some bruising and swelling, possibly obstructing the free flow of urine, a situation known to promote infection."

In addition, a study reported in the *Journal of the American Medical Association* says that women who use a spermicidal jelly or foam are "strongly predisposed" to developing *E. coli* bacteria infections. The researchers believe that spermicides upset the vaginal defense mechanism, so that unfriendly bacteria survive to make the short trip to the bladder. They also point out that diaphragm and spermicide use may contribute to a third of UTIs.

Poor Voiding Habits ▶ Waiting too long before voiding causes the bladder to overfill. This gradually weakens the bladder so that it can't contract with enough force to expel all the urine it's collected. This increases the potential for lingering germs to take up permanent residence in your bladder.

Menopause ▶ As estrogen levels wane, urethra and bladder tissues become thinner and more sensitive to irritation and infection, says Dr. Whitmore. What's more, over time, the bladder naturally loses elasticity and its ability to empty completely.

Targeting the Cause

The good news is that each one of those contributing factors can be countered. In postmenopausal women, for example, estrogen replacement therapy may help turn the tide on cystitis. Sometimes just a topical application of estrogen cream to the vaginal area is all that's needed, says Dr. Whitmore.

"For women who have a known history of urinary tract infections after sexual relations, we now recommend taking one antibiotic tablet just before or after intercourse," she adds. "If the problem seems to stem from diaphragm and spermicide use, we suggest trying another form of birth control, such as a cervical cap. Often, that may end or gradually curtail the problem."

If, despite these preventive measures, infections continue to disrupt your life, long-term prophylaxis is often advised. It's called low-dose suppressive therapy. "We've found that one antibiotic pill every other night can often keep women completely free from infection. After a period of time, we may tell them to discontinue their medication and see what happens," says Dr. Mulholland.

A study by Walter Stamm, M.D., and his colleagues at the University of Washington School of Medicine in Seattle found that low-dose antibiotics, taken for as long as five years, reduced the number of recurrent infections with minimal side effects.

IN THE LADIES' ROOM

Women prone to recurrent bacterial infections may do well to heed the following precautions.

• Take time to empty your bladder completely. When you think you're done urinating, bend over and push forward over your bladder area. Then stand up, sit down, and repeat the maneuver.

• Practice timed toileting. Holding urine too long or trying to void too frequently can both cause problems. Ideally, you should urinate every three to four hours. So schedule your trips to the ladies' room accordingly.

• Wipe from front to back to prevent contaminating the bladder with *E. coli* bacteria from the colon. Take along personal wipes for those occasions when you need to clean yourself away from home.

• Change sanitary napkins or tampons frequently to minimize bacteria growth.

For women who get repeated attacks at random, some doctors encourage self-medication. "We educate the women about the antibiotics, and they keep a stock of them at home," explains Dr. Mulholland. "At the first sign of an infection they can begin a short course of medication. That eliminates time spent phoning the physician, waiting for a callback, going to the office, getting another prescription filled and so forth. These women know when an infection is starting, and this way they can begin medication that much sooner. They keep a medical diary and know what signs or symptoms still require a visit to the doctor. It helps put women back in control of their own bodies."

To check if it's an infection causing your symptoms, there's a home test—as simple as dipping a specially treated test strip into a urine sample and matching its color against a standard.

Bacteria-Free?

Suppose your recurrent bladder problem doesn't fit the standard profile—are no bacteria present in your urine?

Don't be too quick to rule out a bacterial infection. Dr. Stamm and his colleagues say that the criteria used to determine a "positive" urine culture are not sensitive enough. About one-third of women with symptoms of UTI have bacterial counts below the level used to define an infection by laboratory standards. In other words, you can have symptoms even with a small number of bacteria, so small that the laboratory may classify your urine as "normal." Doctors should encourage their laboratory to adopt techniques that detect and report smaller numbers of bacteria, says Dr. Stamm. Dr. Whitmore says your doctor can even request a report on "any bacteria present."

Of course, it's possible that the symptoms you're feeling are not related to an infection after all. "There are a number of possible explanations for this condition, but the most common one is, 'We don't know,'" admits Linda Brubaker, M.D., director of the section of urogynecology at Rush Presbyterian–St. Luke's Medical Center in Chicago. "The discomfort is real enough, though, so we go ahead and treat the symptoms as best we can, while we look for a possible cause.

"Usually, I spend the first two or three visits re-educating the women and proving to them that they do not have an infection," states Dr. Brubaker. "They find it so hard to believe that those symptoms could be present without germs, even though they are persistently culture-negative. Then we start to look at the things in their life that could be exacerbating their symptoms. And this is just trial and error. We don't have scientific evidence that anything makes a difference."

Further research is being funded by the National Institutes of Health. Anything that might irritate the bladder is considered, including the following factors.

Diet ▸ What you eat may be one of the biggest contributors of all, according to the latest opinions from the medical community. Certain foods may irritate the bladder lining in sensitive people. Coffee, wine, chocolate and acidic foods, such as tomatoes and citrus fruits, are the most common offenders. Ironically, foods that may help prevent bacterial infections (including cranberry juice) may contribute to nonbacterial bladder inflammation.

"I've found that patients who have persisted in eating foods to acidify the urine can develop chronic inflammatory bladder disorder," says Dr. Brubaker. "Anecdotally, I

DIET FOR A HEALTHY URINARY TRACT

Perhaps the single most important measure you can take to prevent urinary tract infections (UTIs), and speed your recovery from them, is to drink lots of water—about six to eight eight-ounce glasses a day. Keeping yourself well hydrated helps flush errant bacteria out of your bladder.

Beyond drinking water, however, the diet/cystitis connection is a controversial one. Evidence is sketchy. Doctors, for the most part, remain divided.

Take cranberry juice as an example. Touted for years as a folk cure for UTIs, it was thought to acidify the urine, creating a less hospitable environment for bacteria. Recently, researchers found that a naturally occurring substance found in cranberry juice prevents bacteria from adhering to bladder walls. This may explain how cranberry juice might help prevent bacterial bladder infections.

But there's something else about cranberry juice that has other doctors urging restraint. Some experts now believe that acidifying your urine with cranberry juice during a bladder infection may actually slow down improvement, especially since the bladder is already irritated. Indeed, some liken it to pouring salt on a wound. These experts recommend neutralizing your urine with a low-acid diet, including antacids, watermelon or a glass of water mixed probably get about a 60 percent improvement rate in these patients by taking them off all acidic foods."

Stress ▶ "For some women, especially those in high-pressure positions, the bladder can be used as an end organ for stress. That doesn't mean it's all in your head," cautions Dr. Mulholland. For some, stress expresses itself as bladder symptoms just as for others it might be ulcers

---

with a teaspoon of baking soda two times a day.

Since science has yet to give definitive answers to all this, the best bet for those who believe that diet may exacerbate a flare-up is to try an elimination diet. This involves eliminating the following foods from your diet, then adding them back slowly, one every three days or so. If your condition worsens after the addition of a particular food, you can try avoiding it for extended periods.

• Caffeine-containing foods: coffee, tea, chocolate, colas. (Remember, some drugs contain caffeine.)

• Cranberry and guava juices

• Citrus fruits, along with apples, cantaloupe, grapes, peaches, pineapples, plums, strawberries and tomatoes

• Spicy foods

• Beverages: alcoholic and carbonated

• Vinegars

• Foods that contain the amino acids tyrosine, tyramine, tryptophan and aspartate. They include aspartame, avocados, bananas, beer, cheese, chicken livers, chocolate, corned beef, lima beans, mayonnaise, nuts, onions, prunes, raisins, rye bread, saccharin, sour cream, soy sauce and yogurt.

or migraines. "When I detect that a patient's symptoms may be related to stress, I recommend biofeedback and other stress-reduction techniques," he says.

Menopause ▸ When estrogen levels begin to taper off, urethra and bladder tissues become thinner and more sensitive to irritation.

Chemical Irritants ▸ Soaps and bubble baths can deposit irritating chemicals that work their way into the urinary tract. These irritants can be especially problematic in women whose bladder tissues have become overly sensitized, such as those past menopause.

Sexual Intercourse ▸ Even in the absence of bacteria, the motion of the penis can irritate bladder tissue, causing cystitis-like symptoms. Also, the latex in condoms and diaphragms—as well as the chemicals in spermicides—can cause allergic reactions in some women.

"The bottom line is that these bladder problems sometimes wax and wane over time," says Dr. Brubaker. "And while you may not be able to cure them, you can empower women and give them some control over their symptoms, whether their condition is infectious in nature or bacteria-free."

12   The Eyes Have It

What to look for when buying new glasses.

These days, buying prescription eyeglasses can be every bit as challenging as picking out a new car. Forget simply handing the scribbled prescription to someone in a white coat and choosing a frame that fits nicely on the nose. We're now faced with considerable (and often confusing) options, such as edge treatments, high-index plastic, gradient tints, photochromics, polycarbonates and progressive addition. At least when you shop for a car, you get to take a test drive and kick the tires.

Buyer be wary: You can make shopping for lenses easier on yourself if you're prepared. Whether you obtain your next pair of glasses from a private optician or optometrist or that flashy, super optical chain at the mall, it pays to be armed to the eyes with the latest eyewear information. Some of the available options may make your life easier, but others may just make your wallet lighter. Take a look.

Lens Material

There's a fairly wide assortment of lens materials to choose from, with each meeting specific needs.

Glass ▶ Glass used to be the most widely used material, and it still provides one of the hardest surfaces of all the lenses. But as the large frames gained popularity and the lighter plastics were introduced, desire for thick and heavy glass began to fade.

"If you have a high-powered prescription, wearing thick glass lenses may be too much weight for your nose to bear," says Irving Bennett, O.D., an optometrist and chairman of the information and data committee for the American Optometric Association. Glass is useful primarily for people who want good photochromics—that is, lenses that get darker outdoors or in bright indoor light—he says.

Plastic ▶ "Plastic lenses are safer, more impact-resistant and much lighter than glass, giving you a more comfortable fit," says Richard Morgenthal of Morgenthal-Frederics Opticians, Inc., in New York City. When large lenses became fashionable, lightweight plastic came to dominate the market, forcing glass out to the periphery of lenswear sales.

A plastic lens is more vulnerable to scratches, however. "That's why you should always get a scratch-resistant coating on your plastic lens," says Dr. Bennett. Some

125

places may offer the coating as standard with plastic lenses.

Polycarbonate Plastic ▶ This lens is made of a lighter but tougher plastic—unique enough that eye-care specialists classify it in a separate category.

The polycarbonate plastic lens was first introduced as virtually unbreakable, with people slamming hammers on them to show off their strength. Experts say most people don't really need this kind of protection. Polycarbonate is recommended for children under age 16 and anyone who plays contact sports or who works in a hazardous industry.

Polycarbonate suffers from a few drawbacks as well: It's more prone to scratching (so it has to have that scratch-resistant coating), and it can't be "edged" as well—referring to a method of treating the edge of a lens so it appears even and smooth.

It has a higher index of refraction (meaning it can bend light more than regular plastic), however, so the lens can do more with less material. Thus, it can be made thinner than glass, a plus on the side of cosmetics and comfort.

Coatings and Filters

While coatings are becoming an increasingly popular extra, the real need for some may be overstated. Like light bulbs and toasters, they don't last forever. Their life span can stretch anywhere from six months to two years and up. Most opticians agree that if you take really good care of them, clean them carefully and don't wipe them on your shirttail, coatings can last a few years. Some companies guarantee their coatings for one year or more, sometimes even for the life of the lens.

Scratch-Resistant Coatings ▶ Despite the name, these aren't totally scratchproof, but they do protect against hairline scratches that can occur from cleaning and handling. They won't prevent damage from more serious abuse, such as dropping your lenses on hard pavement, rubbing them against a pen in your pocket or laying them lens-side down. If you're in the habit of doing those things, stop—or getting this coating will be a waste of money.

And if you're buying glass lenses, you won't need this coating. "Glass is hard enough as it is," says Dr. Bennett. "But the coating is necessary for polycarbonate because those lenses are so soft." Scratch-resistant coatings for plastic lenses, he says, are optional and depend on, again, how you treat them.

Tints ► You'd be surprised at the array of tints available to the average eyeball. "Teak," "pecan," "jade" and "charcoal" are just a colorful handful of the latest fashion tints you can add to your lenses. But beyond the cosmetic, is there any reason to get them?

A tint may help give you clearer vision in sunlight, says Morgenthal, especially if you choose brown, green and gray. If you don't want to tint the whole lens, a gradient tint covering only the upper part of the lens may do. You can also split a lens into two tints—one half brown and the other gray, for example. Some outfits do charge for tinting, with whole or partial tints at varying prices, while other places may not charge at all.

UV Filters ► News reports alarm us about possible harm from ultraviolet rays coming from a variety of sources, including holes in the ozone layer. So UV protection has become a big seller at most eye-care outlets. For a fee, the specialist can apply an uncolored coating of protection to keep out UV rays.

Some studies have suggested that UV light is indeed dangerous to the eye. One study of over 800 watermen found high sun exposure was significantly related to increased incidence of cataracts. In other research, sunlight exposure has been linked to cancer of the uveal tract (the most common form of primary eye cancer in adults) and other types of eye cancer. So we know the sun's rays can mean serious business to eye health.

And you should be especially cautious if you've had cataract surgery—in which the eye's lens is removed,

127
∎

exposing the retina—or if you spend a lot of time out-doors or live at high altitudes (where the sun's rays are stronger). Does that mean the UV-coating option is a must to fight the sun? Not exactly.

Most glasses these days already come with UV pro-tection. "Even more, the majority of UV light is filtered by any glass or plastic material," says H. Jay Wisnicki, M.D., director of ophthalmology at Beth Israel Medical Center in New York City. "The extra coatings may not be that important." Take the windows of your car, for exam-ple. If you drive with your arm against the window in the blistering sun, it won't get burned. But hang it out the window and you may get a "truck-driver's tan." That's the kind of protection you get with most glass. So if you want extra peace of mind, you can opt for the coating, but it's not really needed, says Dr. Wisnicki.

As for UV rays seeping from computers, that threat, too, may be exaggerated. "The amount of UV light that comes from a computer is very small and shouldn't be regarded as a problem," says Dr. Wisnicki. The American Academy of Ophthalmology considers video display ter-minals (VDTs) to be completely safe, presenting no haz-ard to the eye. According to the group's latest statement on the subject, "There's no convincing experimental or epidemiologic evidence that exposure to VDTs results in cataracts or any other organic damage to the eye. When people complain of eye problems after using terminals, more likely it's due to eyestrain and an uncomfortable work setting," says Dr. Wisnicki.

Instead, they might rearrange their workspace by adjusting the lighting and screen distance. Remember, too, that glasses made for reading may not help at a com-puter terminal.

Normal reading distance is 16 inches, while a com-puter screen is viewed at 21 inches. That may be forcing the peepers to strain extra hard. There, a specific pre-scription that targets the terminal would help, either as separate glasses or as part of a bifocal.

128

Photochromic Lenses ▶ Photochromics, lenses that change from clear to dark, may be a convenient choice for someone whose job requires a combination of indoor and outdoor work. Different brands go from light when indoors to varying degrees of darkness when outside. "They shouldn't be used for driving, however, because the lenses need UV light to stimulate darkening, and UV light is blocked by windshield glass," says Morgenthal.

If you have photochromics, here's a cool tip to make them work better: "If you consistently store these lenses overnight in the fridge, in general they'll respond quicker to light and get darker," says Morgenthal.

The photochromic option comes primarily in glass. A new type is now made of plastic. But you may still want to stick to glass. Experts say that the earlier plastic prototypes would last about six months and then turn yellow and stay that way. The new version has improved somewhat, but not enough to supersede glass.

Antireflective Coatings ▶ This coating—made from the same material used to coat camera lenses and binoculars—serves two different purposes: to block out reflected glare and also to eliminate the shine that appears on the lens that may hinder the way you look. Not everybody needs this coating, but specific instances occur where it may come in handy.

If you're looking at a bare light bulb without the antireflective coating, you may see two of them. The coating cuts that out and helps to eliminate seeing your own eyeball or eyelashes in the back of your lens. Night drivers may want to steer toward this coating. It virtually eliminates the starburst effect you get from oncoming headlights. It can also cut glare from other types of lighting.

Antireflective coatings (also called antiglare coatings) may also help from the opposite end—influencing what people see when they look at you. If you're in the public eye, this coat may help eliminate the reflections of light that appear on your lens and block out your eyes. If you're watching a bespectacled newscaster on TV and you can see his eyes clearly, chances are his lenses have been treated with the antiglare coating.

One of the bugaboos with antiglare coating, though,

is its tendency to smudge a lot. You'll have to take extra care to keep your lenses clean. Dr. Wisnicki, who owns a pair, agrees, saying, "The dirt seems to show up more." There's a new Teflon coating out now, though, that goes over the antiglare coating and may make it easier to care for the lenses.

Focal Fighters

Previously, when it came to combating presbyopia (the gradual decline in the eye lens's ability to focus on nearby objects), one could turn only to bifocals. With them, only two distances mattered—near and far. There was no in-between. Now new lenses offer effective alternatives to the split-level world of bifocal vision, some erasing the bifocals' age-giveaway lines while giving sharp vision at different distances.

Trifocals ▶ Bifocals have the "near" and "far" covered. If you need to scan a terminal beyond normal reading distance, however, missing that middle distance between near and far means an eyeball of trouble. A trifocal offers that extra area of power on the lens to bridge the near and far. The visual breakdown when looking through a common trifocal lens goes like this: far distance up top, medium distance in the middle and close at the bottom.

Trifocals aren't for everyone. "Some people may not be able to get used to the 'image jumps' that occur when switching from one segment to the next," says Richard E. Lippman, O.D., director of the division of ophthalmic devices for the Food and Drug Administration. It's a problem encountered with bifocals and can become more troublesome in a trifocal with the extra segment, he says.

"Unless your work really calls for a specific middle distance, I wouldn't really prescribe a trifocal," says Dr. Wisnicki. That's why an eye-care professional should take a complete history of your lifestyle and occupation. If you find that your daily activities really require using all three vision segments, then trifocals may be a viable option.

Progressive-Addition Lenses ▸ If the bifocal or trifocal is the stairway of lenses, then a progressive bifocal
lens is the smooth ramp. Gone are the abrupt jumps in
vision power. Instead, you see a blended transition from
one segment of vision to the next. It's a smooth swim
from top to bottom, closely mimicking natural, good
vision.

The most obvious benefit the progressive-addition
lenses have over bifocals is the absence of the age-telling
line. "The line can't be seen because the focal powers
blend into each other," says Dr. Bennett.

The powers blend together this way: Distance is at
the top, intermediate is in the middle, and reading is
at the bottom. Some people may be able to use these
lenses like trifocals—looking through the center por-
tion to view middle distances, like computer screens
that are an arm's length away. Unlike trifocals, small
areas of distortion exist off to the sides, out of your
direct line of vision.

Some people have trouble getting used to these glasses, while others don't. "Some eyes adapt better to the
visual conditions and the minor distortion than others,"
Dr. Bennett says.

It may depend on your eye-care history. "The more
complex or difficult your prescription is before you need
bifocals, the more distortion you will already have off to
the sides," says Dr. Bennett. "So people who have strong
prescriptions find it easiest to get used to progressive-
addition lenses." Someone who's never had bifocals may
take to these lenses easier than someone who's been
wearing bifocals for years. The seasoned bifocal wearer
may be uncomfortable at first with the new blend, whereas a first-time bifocal wearer has nothing to compare the
progressives with. "As much as I like this lens, I won't
automatically switch a patient with bifocals to progressives," says Dr. Wisnicki. "But if they say they're having
trouble seeing at that intermediate distance, between the
near and far of the bifocal powers, I strongly suggest the
progressive lens."

To get progressive-addition lenses to work best takes
several precise measurements. If the measurements are

off, you may end up looking into the distortion.

Motivation is also key when it comes to getting used to these lenses. You need to work them in, like a new pair of shoes. "For some people, it may take a few hours to get used to the lens; for others it may take days, weeks, even longer," says Dr. Wisnicki. "But if you stick it out for a while, in time the lenses should present no problem, and you'll actually start to like them."

Says Penny Asbell, M.D., associate professor of ophthalmology at Mount Sinai Medical Center in New York City, "Try to get some kind of guarantee in case you find them unsuitable." Most manufacturers offer such deals.

Plus, if the lenses do present a problem, at the very least you can take them back and have them checked. It may have been an incorrect measurement that's causing a problem. Any reputable outfit will check, remeasure and replace faulty lenses.

"For people who need to see at close range and from side to side, like an architect working with wide blueprints, it may not be the best choice," says Morgenthal. The areas of vision may be too narrow for them.

"And the distortion may seem odd at first, but the fact is you really don't use that part of the lens," says Dr. Wisnicki. "Rarely do you read or look at an object with your eyes shifting back and forth to each corner," he says. And new lenses continue to come out that reduce the distorted areas.

If you don't want a progressive lens, you can try "hidden-line" bifocals. These lenses have a blurred line dividing near and far vision, which can only be seen from the side. And there is one other potential solution in tackling the distance between near and far. Get another pair of glasses dealing specifically with that distance and keep them handy.

If your job requires you to focus at one distance for a long period, your optometrist can provide you with lenses geared for that chore. Even more, special bifocals can be made that reverse the location of the focal powers, with the near vision up top and far on bottom. That may be a wise choice for someone who paints ceilings and needs to see things above him up close.

KEEPING THEM CLEAN

No doubt you've heard a number of suggestions on how to keep your lenses spotless. Here's the wash, from our experts.

• "By far the best cleaning solution is soap and water," says Irving Bennett, O.D., an optometrist and chairman of the information and data committee for the American Optometric Association. "Clean your lenses with a nonabrasive soap and then dry with a fine, soft cloth or paper towel."

"You can't bring the kitchen sink with you, but try washing with a mild liquid detergent, rinsing with warm water. Then lightly blot with a good-quality paper towel," adds Richard Morgenthal, of Morgenthal-Frederics Opticians, Inc., in New York City. "The soap immediately dissolves and lifts off anything that would have an oily base to it, such as sweat or makeup."

Be careful with the new cleaning sprays on the market. "Picture a lens that has some dust and dirt on it," says Morgenthal. "By spritzing it with a cleaner and then rubbing it with a soft hanky, you are grinding that abrasive dust into the surface of the lens," he says.

• Beware of bars. "Hand soaps leave an oily film on antireflective-coated lenses, especially if they contain lanolin, and it's difficult to remove," says Morgenthal. Some tissues contain softeners that also leave a film.

• Don't wipe your lenses dry or you'll scratch them up. One exception: "There are some very closely knit cloths in the market today that allow you to clean the lenses dry," says Dr. Bennett. They cost about $3 to $5 and can be picked up at your local optical shop.

• When you clean plastic lenses, first run them under water, using the pressure from the tap to rinse away grit. Beware of hot water—it can stretch a plastic frame, says Morgenthal.

Anti-Thick Tricks

Here are some options for those who need strong prescription glasses but don't want the "Coke-bottle" look or a heavy load on the nose.

High Index ▸ A high-index lens is simply a denser lens with a higher power of refraction, meaning it can bend more light than the standard-index glasses, so less material is needed to do the job. Thus the lens can be thinner and therefore lighter.

"I suggest high-index lenses to just about everyone with high prescriptions who would otherwise have to wear very thick glass or thick ordinary plastic lenses," says Dr. Wisnicki.

High index is more expensive and has one other disadvantage, called chromatic aberration.

"This occurs more at night," says Dr. Wisnicki. "You may see blue halos around headlights and streetlights. If you look straight through the center of the lens at an object, though, the streaks and halos markedly decrease." Since you're essentially looking through a prism when wearing these eyeglasses, colors abound. "Blue is the most noticeable one," says Dr. Wisnicki, "but again the benefits of a much thinner lens may outweigh this insignificant problem."

The amount that lens thickness can be reduced by switching to high index depends upon the prescription. "The stronger the prescription, the more pronounced an effect the high index has on thickness," says Dr. Wisnicki. So the people who need it most are helped the most.

"If you have a low prescription, though, the change won't be so great," he adds. There, high index may be unnecessary—the thickness won't be reduced as much, and you'll still be paying a higher price.

The high-index eyeglass can improve the appearance of large-area lenses, making them thinner. If the lenses are cut smaller, however, to fit a John Lennon–style frame, for example, the difference in thickness will be less.

Edge Treatments ▶ Some optical stores offer ways to hide the telltale thickness of a powerful lens.

In a special edging process called "hide-a-bevel," an eye-care specialist polishes and shaves the edges down to take away that abrupt cut of a thick lens. You may also be able to get an enamel coating placed on the edges of lenses that matches the color and texture of the frame.

"Because you don't see a white edge of the lens, you can't see how thick the lens is," says Morgenthal. And the thicker the lens is originally, the more these techniques help.

Antireflective Coatings and Tints ▶ Aside from the other benefits mentioned earlier, both these extras may

---

MAKE THE RIGHT EYE CONTACT

Ophthalmologist, optometrist, optician—can you tell the difference? They all deal with eyeballs and wear white coats, but big differences exist among them.

Ophthalmologists. These are eye surgeons and physicians who carry an M.D. or D.O. at the end of their name. They specialize in the diagnosis and treatment of eye disease. They can also give vision tests and prescribe glasses and contact lenses.

Optometrists. They aren't M.D.'s but state-licensed professionals who check visual function and also treat nonsurgical eye problems. Often when they detect problems, such as eye disease, they can refer the patient to an ophthalmologist. They also prescribe glasses and contact lenses. In 28 states, they're licensed to prescribe medications and manage certain eye diseases.

Opticians. These professionals fill prescriptions for eyeglasses and in some states can do the same for contact lenses. They can only fill prescriptions generated by ophthalmologists and optometrists. In only 26 states are opticians required to be licensed in order to practice.

135

help slim the appearance of a lens. "The antireflective coating may reduce the concentric circles you see when you look at someone with thick lenses," says Morgenthal. And a tint may enhance the look of the lenses, especially thick ones, by softening their appearance.

13 New Treatments for Fibroids

Hysterectomy is no longer the only option.

Elsa Davidson, a 45-year-old nutritionist, discovered she had uterine fibroids several years ago during a routine gynecological examination. Although her doctor said she was "filled with them," they had caused her no discomfort. So she did as her doctor suggested: kept tabs on their growth with yearly checkups.

But during those five years the fibroids grew steadily. She knew decision time was drawing near when the fibroids became so large that they began pushing on her bladder, causing occasional incontinence. After more discussions with her doctor, she decided that a hysterectomy was the right choice for her.

Does this story sound familiar? It's probably the kind of scenario that many women envision when they consider what happens when someone gets fibroids. And indeed, Elsa's story is typical. But hysterectomy is not the only option—now there are newer uterus-saving treatments to consider.

The Do-Nothing-Now Option

Fibroids are tumors composed mostly of muscle tissue, ranging in size from a pea to a cantaloupe or larger. They can be outside or inside the uterus, embedded in the uterine walls or attached by stalks (pedunculated fibroids). Nobody really knows why they appear in the first place, but they do in about 20 to 25 percent of women over 35.

They're rarely cancerous—only about 1 in 1,000 is. So if you have no symptoms there may be no reason to take action, says Ruth Schwartz, M.D., clinical professor of obstetrics and gynecology at the University of Rochester School of Medicine, in Rochester, New York.

Since fibroids depend on estrogen for their growth, a woman nearing menopause (a time when estrogen production begins to decline) may be able to "wait out" her fibroids. The growths are likely to shrink or disappear after menopause. For younger women, it's best to monitor fibroids to see if they grow, how fast and whether they start to cause major discomfort, says Dr. Schwartz. Fibroid size and growth rates are monitored during annual pelvic exams by a woman's doctor actually feeling them or by ultrasound.

The American College of Obstetricians and Gynecologists (ACOG) says that about a third of women with fibroids complain of heavy bleeding with their periods. Another third experience pressure and pelvic pain.

Fibroids can also interfere with pregnancy and delivery, although admittedly the vast majority of pregnant patients with fibroids have no trouble at all, says Carol Ann Burton, M.D., clinical instructor of obstetrics and gynecology at the University of Southern California in Los Angeles.

"If a fibroid is located on the inside of the uterus, the placenta may not implant properly, leading to a first-trimester miscarriage," she says. "Sometimes, fibroids grow rapidly during pregnancy due to the hormonal environment. As the uterus stretches, premature labor may occur. Or the fibroid may outgrow its blood supply and die, causing excruciating pain as it degenerates. Women may be advised to have them removed if subsequent pregnancies are planned."

"Traditional" Myomectomy

To remove fibroids, you don't have to remove the whole uterus. Believe it or not, the first myomectomy (surgical removal of fibroids) was performed in the late 1800s, says Andrew J. Friedman, M.D., associate professor of obstetrics, gynecology and reproductive biology at Harvard Medical School. And what could be called the "traditional" myomectomy is getting to be more popular— perhaps because more women are demanding alternatives to hysterectomy, especially if they want to have children. Each year about 18,000 of these procedures are performed.

During a traditional myomectomy a physician makes an abdominal incision, then an incision in the uterus. The fibroids are cut out, then the incisions are stitched closed. The abdominal incision is usually four to six inches long.

This type of myomectomy may be the answer for many, since it's a way of removing troublesome tumors while still leaving the uterus in place. Not that this procedure is free of drawbacks. Like any major surgery, there's the possibility for blood loss requiring blood transfusion, infection or an adverse reaction to anesthesia. In fact, blood loss may be even greater for this than hysterectomy, although recuperation time is about the same—four to six weeks. What's more, in about 25 percent of cases the fibroids regrow within five years, either from little "seedlings" that were missed during the initial surgery or from new fibroids that developed since the operation. Then the operation may have to be repeated, or a hysterectomy done after all. And the more fibroids you have, the greater your chance of recurrence.

Because the surgeon is cutting into the uterus, there can be scarring that may cause problems with pregnancy or fertility later. These complications, however, are rare. And for women whose fibroids are causing pregnancy problems, the operation is usually beneficial. These women need to understand, though, that when they do get pregnant, they may have to deliver by cesarean section because the uterine walls have been weakened.

Microsurgery

If you have very small fibroids, you may be eligible for some of the newer myomectomies that shorten recuperation time as well as reduce complications.

Fibroids that extend into the cavity of the uterus, for example, may be handled with a hysteroscope, a tele-scope-type instrument that's inserted through the vagina and cervix, allowing visual inspection of the inside of the uterus. Depending on the technique your doctor is most skilled with, the hysteroscope can be equipped with a laser that burns away the tumors or with an instrument that shaves down the tumors, called a resectoscope. With this technique, an electric current is run through a horse-shoe-shaped wire, which shaves off the growths layer by layer.

Small fibroids that are located on the outside of the uterus, on the other hand, can often be removed with the use of a laparoscope, another telescope-type instrument, which is inserted through a tiny incision near the navel. It allows visual inspection of the outside of the uterus. The laparoscope can be equipped with a laser or other cauterizing attachment to remove fibroids.

Both the hysteroscopic and laparoscopic procedures are done on an outpatient basis, a major advantage. The procedures themselves cost about the same as a tradi-tional myomectomy, but generally there are no hospital costs. There may be mild cramping for a few days after-ward, Dr. Schwartz says, but recovery is quick, and you can usually return to work in less than a week. The downside is that even with these less invasive proce-dures, the tumors may still grow back, necessitating a possible repeat performance or a hysterectomy.

Shrink First, Operate Later

Even if your fibroids are large, you may still take advantage of microsurgical techniques. New drugs—called GnRH agonists—taken for a few months can shrink fibroids down to a small enough size that major abdominal surgery can sometimes be avoided.

These drugs block the production of estrogen from the ovaries. And since fibroids are estrogen-sensitive tumors, they shrink when it's no longer available—by 40 to 50 percent on average. And because they cut down the

139
∎

blood supply in the uterus, says Dr. Schwartz, myomectomies can be performed with less blood loss.

Actually, if you should happen to be near menopause, taking one of these drugs may help you eliminate surgery altogether, says Dr. Burton. By the time you finish a course of treatment, your own body's natural decline in estrogen production may finish the job for you.

Now for the downside. The two drugs with approval from the Food and Drug Administration (FDA)—nafarelin acetate (administered via nasal spray) and leuprolide acetate (given by injection)—don't come cheap. They run $250 to $400 per month, says Dr. Friedman, and some insurance companies may not cover the expense, since these drugs are still considered experimental. The drugs are approved by the FDA for endometriosis but not for fibroids, though doctors do use them for this purpose. And they can be taken safely for only six months. Shutting down your estrogen production puts you into an artificial menopause and at risk for developing the bone-thinning disease osteoporosis.

Also, if you stop taking these drugs, and if your own estrogen kicks in again, the fibroids may start to grow again, usually within six months. That may not matter if the idea is to shrink the fibroids enough for microsurgery.

Doctors recognize the potential benefits of being able to use GnRH agonists for longer periods of time, though, and are working on eliminating their negative aspects. Dr. Friedman is experimenting with GnRH in combination with a low dose of estrogen and progesterone. "The idea is to give enough estrogen to counteract menopausal side effects, such as hot flashes and the potential for osteoporosis," he says, "but a low enough dose so you don't cause a regrowth of the fibroid. So far, it appears to work well for some women, but not so well for others."

Halting a Fibroid Symptom

If your fibroids are not large, and the only grief they're giving you is heavy bleeding, there are other options.

Drugs such as danazol or high-dose progestins can often curb abnormally heavy bleeding, although they'll do nothing to shrink the fibroids. You may, however, find that the side effects are more than you care to live with. About 80 percent of women get some side effects, which include excess weight gain, bloating, hair growth, elevated cholesterol and vaginal spotting. These are mild in most cases.

Another alternative is a procedure called laser ablation therapy, developed 12 years ago by Milton Goldrath, M.D., chief of gynecology at Sinai Hospital in Detroit, Michigan. Using a laser-equipped hysteroscope, the uterine lining is literally destroyed. No lining, no bleeding. But your fibroids are still there and could conceivably grow and give you trouble. "You're also considered sterile after this procedure," he says. "So, clearly, this isn't for everyone. If you've completed your family, however, have a uterus that's not larger than the size of a 12-week pregnancy and the heavy bleeding cannot be controlled by other means, then laser ablation is a possible solution."

It's done on an outpatient basis, and recovery is very quick, says Dr. Goldrath. "Patients go home the same day and are back to work in just one or two days." Side effects are usually mild.

Your Own Best Choice

There's no one treatment that's just right for everyone. As Dr. Friedman points out, "You need to be clear about your goals. Have you had three miscarriages? Do you just want to stop excessive bleeding or control it better? Are your fibroids so large that you look pregnant? Are they pressing on your bladder, causing frequent urination?

"In other words," he says, "what do you hope to achieve from your treatment? Whatever it is, make that very clear to your doctor. Question him or her about what is being planned and why. Seek a second opinion if you feel uncertain about the doctor's judgment or simply want more information. You may feel that a hysterectomy is the right choice for you. It is, after all, the only sure 'cure' for fibroids. In any case, look for a doctor skilled in the technique that you've decided upon."

141

The Power of Exercise

Worry-Free Walking   14

How to keep your feet moving despite nature's obstacles.

True, walking is a pretty carefree exercise. The kinds of things that distract you often don't seem bothersome enough to find a solution. But why let a few unpleasant details or fears spoil your enjoyment of a summer walk?

Here is a list of some common "walking gremlins," and some suggestions for preventing them.

Swollen Hands

You step out for a brisk walk, and after 15 minutes or so, your hands feel like balloons. They're red, puffy and—if you have on any rings—choking! As long as this swelling occurs only when you walk, it's just the centrifugal force of your arm movement forcing blood into your hands. For greater comfort, leave your rings at home. If the feeling of swollen hands disturbs you, try walking with your elbows bent for a while. When you stop walking, your hands should resume their former size and shape.

Sudden Storms

Summer showers can come on quickly and without much warning. While the always-prepared types may carry a rain jacket in a pouch, many people will simply get soaked. Problem? Not according to Murray Hamlet, director of the Cold Research Program, U.S. Army Research Institute of Environmental Medicine, Natick, Massachusetts. "If you're not in danger of getting lost and being exposed for a long period of time, getting soaked doesn't put you at risk for hypothermia. Just cover up as best you can and keep walking. The exercise will keep your body warm enough."

Worried about catching a cold? Save your energy.

Wet hair or clothing and raw weather may aggravate existing symptoms, but they won't make you sick, says Richard Clover, M.D., of the University of Oklahoma Health Sciences Center. According to Dr. Clover, when it comes to colds, you should worry more about who you shake hands with than the weather. Colds are caused by viruses, which are often transmitted by something as simple as a handshake.

If the sudden storm includes lightning, beware of standing under isolated trees, in open fields, near tractors or heavy equipment or near water. Those are the places where most people in the United States have been hit (1,953 people were killed between 1959 and 1987). Thirty-one were killed at telephones. If you find yourself in a wide-open space with thunder booming and daggers of lightning slashing the skies, don't lie flat on the ground. Drop to your knees, bend forward, and put your hands on your knees.

If a storm is brewing and you literally feel your hair stand on end, a close hit may be imminent. Take precautions. Lightning can hit miles from the parent cloud. Find the lowest spot or shelter under a group of trees, not an isolated one. If you're walking with a group, spread out. You'll be less of a target.

Angry Dogs

During the summer months, many dogs are allowed outside by owners who aren't aware that their friendly house pet may become a snarling wolf dog around strangers. But dogs are territorial, and they often learn to consider the sidewalk and street around their home as their turf. In fact, that's where most bites occur.

Don't ever underestimate the viciousness of a strange dog. According to Alan Beck, Sc.D., director of the Center for Applied Ethology and Human-Animal Interaction at Purdue University School of Veterinary Medicine, most bites occur with people who have their own pets or had them as children. They assume they can approach a strange animal.

If you can avoid areas where you know dogs are loose,

do that. Or you may want to call the local authorities and find out what the leash laws are and report violations. If you do come face-to-face with a strange dog, avoid eye contact. It's seen as a challenge by the dog. If the dog's ears and hackles (the fur along the back of his neck and back) are up, if he is growling or baring his teeth, slowly back off. If he persists in coming toward you, yell at him: "Go home!" Put something between you and the dog. Offer a stick or even a cassette player, rather than your hand or arm, for protection. A commercial dog repellent can be very effective. Don't be afraid to use it.

If you happen to be walking your own dog and you see a stray dog coming, turn around and walk the other way. If a fight does ensue, stay out of it, or you'll most likely get bitten. Try distraction. Throw something at them—your hat, stick, cap. According to Dr. Beck, a water pistol often works. It's the next best thing to the old bucket-of-water trick.

Pesky Yellow Jackets

Ever wonder why yellow jackets seem to be dive-bombing you with more tenacity toward the end of the summer? According to Peter J. Landolt, Ph.D., an entomologist with the U.S. Department of Agriculture Laboratory at the University of Florida, the pesky critters are searching for sugar to feed the emerging queens and males in the nest. They are attracted to flowery perfumes, and the color they like best is yellow! Leave that Hawaiian shirt at home!

Don't try to swat them if they're disturbing your peace. If you squash the venom sac, a substance is released that calls in all their buddies for an attack. Just keep walking. Chances are, if they can't find any sugar on you, they'll move on to sweeter pastures.

If you do get stung, be prepared to flee. Yellow jackets can strike again. Head indoors, into water or into the woods. They'll have trouble following you into a thicket.

To deal with the pain out on a walk, a cool stream would be convenient. At home, an ice pack rubbed on the area can prevent the venom from spreading and cut down

145
■

on swelling. If you're allergic to bee stings, they can be dangerous. Carry your insect-sting kit. Symptoms of an allergic reaction to a sting are chest tightness, hives, nausea, vomiting, wheezing, dizziness, swollen tongue or face, fainting or shock. The more rapidly these symptoms appear, the more life-threatening. Have someone take you to an emergency medical service immediately.

Side Stitches

Walking briskly, you suddenly experience a stabbing pain in your side. A torn muscle? A gallbladder attack? Probably not. Side stitches are caused by a spasm of the diaphragm, a muscle between your chest and your abdomen. The muscle is crying out for oxygen because your expanded lungs and contracted abdomen are blocking normal blood flow. Not to worry. Stop walking. Using three fingers, press on the area where the pain is greatest until the hurt stops. Or gently massage the area. Often this is enough to relieve the pain. Don't hold your breath! As your breathing resumes a regular pace, the ache should also subside.

Remember to warm up by walking slowly when you start out. Going too fast too soon can cause your diaphragm to cramp, just like any other muscle that is not warmed up properly.

Shin Splints

You're walking through the park on the nice flat macadam path, heel-and-toeing along, and suddenly the front of your lower leg begins to burn. Or maybe when you got up this morning your shins were sore from yesterday's walk. Nobody is exactly sure what shin splints are, according to Marjorie Albohm, M.S., associate director of the International Institute of Sports Science and Medicine at the Indiana University School of Medicine. But don't worry, we do know what to do about them.

If possible, walk on a soft surface. If you can't change to grass or dirt, try upgrading your shoes. Look for walking shoes with plenty of shock absorption and arch support. After you've done a little slow walking to warm up, stretch your calf muscles, which relieves stress on your shins. Lean against a pole or wall, place one foot back, and gently lower your heel to the ground. Repeat 20 times with each leg.

When pain hits, apply ice and elevate your legs for 20 to 30 minutes.

Sometimes you can avoid shin splints by strengthening the muscles around the shin. One easy way for walkers to do this is to spend some time walking around on their heels. If you've been working out on a stationary bike all winter, you've also been building protection from shin pain.

How do you know when it's not a shin splint but a stress fracture? A fracture has a specific point of pain on or around a bony area, about the size of a dime or quarter. You literally are able to put your finger on it.

Chafing Thighs

Shorts feel great in the summertime, except for one thing. Take away that protective material that long pants provide and sweaty thighs rubbing against each other may cause chafing. Solution? Try rubbing some petroleum jelly on your inner thighs. You'll be protected from moisture and friction.

Bathroom Urgencies

Everybody can identify with the little kid bundled in the snowsuit who tells his mom at the last minute that he has to go to the bathroom. Being a half mile from home can be the summer equivalent of a snowsuit if you're out for a walk and the urge to "go" hits. Don't worry, the first sign of the need to empty your bladder is an early warning signal, according to Lester Klein, M.D., at the Scripps Clinic, Urology Division. That signal usually fades if you keep walking. You've got time to play with. The next time you feel the urge, your body is saying "Hey! Things are getting serious here." And you'd better start heading for home. The third sensor is pain. Don't let things go that far. You have to learn your body's personal limits. Most people can walk for an hour without a problem. If you can't, you may have to make smaller circuits near your home or stop at a restroom facility in a park.

On a hot day, try drinking water an hour or so before your walk, to avoid dehydration. You'll probably be able to empty your bladder of excess water before you walk. If you're going for a short walk, under an hour, rehydrate when you return. If it's going to be more than an hour, take water along and make sure you're able to empty your bladder when you need to.

If you have health problems, check with your doctor before walking outside on a hot day. He may recommend mall-walking. (Bathroom facilities are usually available.)

Sunscreen Sting

To protect your skin, summer and winter, wear a sunscreen. In the summer, when you're more likely to be sweating a lot, sunscreen may rub off or, worse, roll or be rubbed into your eyes. Bring tissues to wipe it away, or wear sweatbands around your forehead and wrists.

Sunscreens may not be harmful to your eyes, but they can create a painful burning sensation. Look for sunscreens that are waterproof or water-resistant. They are less likely to sweat off during a walking workout.

Creative Urges

Walking enhances creativity. That's great, right? When you're out walking, you may be bombarded with wonderful ideas. The quandary is, should you carry a pen and paper to write them down? Can your walk be as stress-reducing if you're busy solving your own or everybody else's problems, or redesigning the kitchen?

According to Robert Thayer, Ph.D., professor of psychology at California State University, Long Beach, and author of *The Biopsychology of Mood and Arousal,* it's probably true that walking puts you in an optimal mood for problem solving. And if that's your goal, by all means, bring paper! However, if you're suffering from anxious thoughts or under a lot of stress, it's probably best, says Dr. Thayer, to leave your paper at home and try to forget your problems. Allow the walk to distract you. Concentrate on the scenery or perhaps your breathing. Allow intruding thoughts to surface, but don't focus on them. In effect, don't worry, keep walking!

Perspiration Protection 15

Don't let sweat put a damper on your day.

Just when you want to feel in control, a telltale trickle undermines your self-confidence. You may be saying "No sweat!" but your armpits say otherwise.

Sweating is an involuntary response, like breathing, and just as normal. "Sweat is absolutely essential," says Norman Levine, M.D., professor and chief of dermatology at the University of Arizona Health Sciences Center. "It's a primary way your body regulates its internal temperature."

As your body heats up—whether from physical or emotional stress—the perspiration output increases to cool you as water evaporates from your skin's surface. Millions of sweat glands work to cool your body, but only the apocrine sweat glands, concentrated in your armpit, genital and—to a lesser degree—breast area, are responsible for body odor. Like the rest of your sweat glands, these produce a clear, odorless fluid.

After puberty, however, the chemical composition of the apocrine sweat includes new compounds. When these new compounds are broken down by the bacteria that live in the dark, protected armpit area, they create the characteristic smell we recognize as body odor.

Simple sweat may be normal, but it's a problem for many people. New products and a better understanding of your body's cooling system can end your perspiration worries.

Counter-Sweat Measures

Many people are concerned that they sweat too much. "People tend to think of sweating 'too much' as any amount of sweat that makes them uncomfortable," says Dr. Levine. "Most of my patients when questioned have a normal amount of sweating but aren't controlling it adequately. For some it's as simple as using an antiperspirant (which is formulated to control perspiration) rather than a plain deodorant (which just protects against odor)."

Most antiperspirants are a basic formulation of aluminum or zinc salts. These are very effective when used correctly and are well tolerated by most people. To be labeled an antiperspirant, a product has to reduce the sweat output by only 20 percent. So if your present product isn't giving you enough protection, it doesn't necessarily mean you sweat abnormally. Switching to a different antiperspirant should solve your problems.

The strongest antiperspirant available without a prescription is 12 percent aluminum chloride. As with any over-the-counter product, it's important to follow the directions. These products should be applied sparingly at night and never immediately after a bath or shower. Do not use one if your skin is broken or irritated, and never after shaving. The final caution is that if applied during the day, it can damage clothing.

Antiperspirants vary in strength not only because of the ingredients but also depending on whether you are using a spray, stick or roll-on. Generally speaking, aerosols give the least protection, and roll-ons the most. In laboratory tests, however, it became apparent that people react quite individually to antiperspirants, so try several before you decide you have a perspiration problem.

Some people do produce an abnormal amount of sweat. This can be determined either by volume (soaking through your blouse or shirt on a regular basis) or by circumstances (profuse sweating even when you're cool and relaxed). In both these cases, consult your dermatologist. Such excessive sweating may require a prescription antiperspirant.

Counter-Odor Tactics

Some people don't sweat much, no matter how stressed they are. However, that does not mean they don't have to worry about body odor. It doesn't take much perspiration to mix with the bacteria and cause body odor—especially when you're nervous.

"Body odor is worse when you're stressed because the apocrine glands react to stress," says George Preti, Ph.D., a member of the Monell Chemical Senses Center and associate professor of dermatology at the University of Pennsylvania. "They're part of the fight-or-flight syndrome. Fear, anger and excitement can all trigger the apocrine glands."

Even if you don't produce a lot more sweat in these circumstances, your apocrine glands may excrete more of the compound that the bacteria create odor from. Deodorants combat body odor not by reducing the sweat but by reducing the number of bacteria present and also by using fragrance to mask the odor. They are basically perfumes that usually contain a mild antibacterial agent. Remember though, deodorants offer no protection against excess sweating.

Preventive Hygiene

Good hygiene is an integral part of staying sweet smelling. For a little extra protection, choose a deodorant soap.

"Antibacterial soaps are one of the most effective means of cutting down on the bacteria count," explains Dr. Levine. "In general, these aren't the beauty bars because the antibacterial agents are too drying—they're the real soaps with a high pH that help reduce the bacteria count but can tend to be irritating." This means using a different cleanser for your face and your body. But if you're concerned about body odor, the trade-off is certainly well worth it.

Not everyone who uses a deodorant wants the scent. An effective product for those folks is a French import, Le Crystal Naturel, which is actually a crystalline rock of

100 percent mineral salts. To use it you simply moisten the rock and rub it gently over your skin. It claims to be hypoallergenic and won't stain clothes.

16   Bone Boosters

Resistance exercises can help build strong bones fast.

While we sit and talk, work and breathe, architects are constantly at work in our bones. Consisting of bone-forming cells (osteoblasts) and bone-removal cells (osteo-clasts), these construction engineers take part in what you might call the Battle of the Bone—a tug-of-war over your skeleton.

Simply put, the bone removers are winning. After you reach maturity, they work faster, stealing up to 4 percent of your bone each year after menopause. Meanwhile, the bone farmers manage to crank out new bone at only a 2 percent rate. The pluses and minuses don't add up in our favor. And too often the result is osteoporosis, the bone-thinning disease that can lead to "spontaneous fractures."

Enter a secret weapon to assist the bone-forming cells and help bring that equation back into balance: resistance training. All-around physical activity can maintain and even increase bone mass. But what can resistance training do for your bones? Cutting-edge research is beginning to suggest that resistance exercis-es—primarily those that target specific osteoporotic hot spots—may actually prevent bone loss and stimulate an increase in bone mass in those vulnerable areas.

Measurable Gains

In one study, pushing exercises using the forearm helped boost bone in that area in a group of 70-year-old osteoporotic women. The women pushed against a wall or clasped their hands together and pushed them against each other in three weekly workouts for five months. They experienced a 3.8 percent increase in bone in the distal radius (wrist), while the nonexercisers saw a decline of 1.9 percent.

"Even in a short period of time, they saw increases in an area of bone where many fractures occur," says Sydney Lou Bonnick, M.D., director of osteoporosis services at the Cooper Clinic in Dallas.

In another study, this time of middle-aged women, exercise helped stave off bone loss that usually accompanies the middle years. The 4-year study included use of light weights and resistance bands to strengthen the upper body. Ten of the 18 areas of bone mass measured showed significantly reduced bone loss among the exercisers. Projected over 20 years, the bone mass of the ulna (the forearm bone on the side of the little finger) normally would decline 25 percent. In the exercise group, that steep decline was projected to tilt up in a big way—slowing to just 5 percent.

Studies of the racket arms of tennis players show a much higher bone mass in that limb than the nonracket arm. "The bone density is greater in that arm simply because it encounters more resistance," says Kenneth H. Cooper, M.D., president and founder of the Institute for Aerobics Research. "Any resistance exercise targeting a bone tends to do that."

Weight-bearing exercises like stair climbing and walking—targeting the lower limbs—have also caused significant increases in bone mass. Small increases in the spine have been shown to occur, even though the resistance exercises used didn't target that crucial zone. These increases (less than 1 percent in a group of 34 women at Texas Woman's University) may be considered insignificant in this 12-month study. But over a sustained period they could add up. Even more, gaining or maintaining bone mass means one simple yet monumental thing—you aren't losing any. In that sense, it's not insignificant that you're slowing—even reversing—one of the so-called inevitables of aging.

Bone experts agree. "Exercise may be the greatest stimulator that bone ever gets and may maintain and even increase your bone mass," says Everett L. Smith,

Ph.D., director of the Biogerontology Laboratory in the Department of Preventive Medicine at the University of Wisconsin. "It may help maintain a younger bone—a younger bone that is more resistant to fracture."

How to Hit the Hot Spots

The hips, spine and wrists are the most vulnerable and most common sites of osteoporotic fractures, with

BONE WORKOUTS

Here are some specific exercises that may improve bone health.

SPINE

1. Back-machine extensions. As you sit, a padded bar rests against your back, shoulder-blade level. The bar offers the resistance, depending on how much weight you have on the machine. Lean back, still seated, pushing the bar backward, arching your back for each repetition.

2. Back floor extensions. Lie flat on your stomach with your arms by your sides and your palms up. Slowly and gently raise your head and shoulders toward the ceiling until you feel a comfortable stretch in your lower back. Keep your hips in contact with the floor as you stretch, with your eyes and head forward. Lower slowly and then repeat. For added strengthening, also raise both legs.

3. Squats. This exercise is more strenuous and should be done slowly and carefully. Concentrate on your form. Place the bar on your upper back, across your shoulders.

Grip the bar comfortably. Keep your head up and your back slightly arched. Squat slowly until your upper thighs are at a 45-degree angle to the floor. Return to starting position. Inhale down, exhale up during each repetition.

hip and spine fractures resulting in the most illness and death. Wrist fractures are obviously much less life-threatening but are often painful and debilitating.

What follows is an exercise program targeted at those flash points of fracture, to prevent these breaks from happening and bone from leaving home. (Remember, though, that exercise is not a substitute for other osteoporosis prevention measures, such as a good diet and proper medical care.)

WRIST AND FOREARM

4. Wrist curl. Hold a weight (one to three pounds for beginners) in one hand, palm up. Sit at the end of a chair, lean forward with your back slightly arched, and place your forearm on your upper thigh. Place the back of your wrist over your knee. Lower the bar as far as you can; curl the weight back toward you. Repeat with your other arm. Rest between sets.

HIP

These use a pulley machine or a stretch band.

5. Hip extension. Stand in front of the wall pulley. With the ankle strap on your right ankle, step back far enough from the pulley so your leg supports the weight stack. Raise your right leg back to the rear as far as possible. Return to starting position. After exercising one leg for eight to ten repetitions, switch to the other leg.

6. Hip abduction. Stand with your left side facing the wall pulley. With the ankle strap on your right ankle, step back far enough from the pulley so that your leg supports the weight stack. Stand with your legs together. Raise your right leg up and out to the side as far as possible. Return to starting position. After eight to ten repetitions, stand with your right side to the wall and repeat with the left leg.

And don't forget the main benefit of resistance training—it builds muscle. By boosting strength, you may reduce the risk of falling and the force of impact if you do. That alone may cut the risk of many osteoporotic fractures. So while you're working the bone, you're also creating and improving upon a fracture-proofing jacket of muscle—one that surrounds your skeleton and provides a cushion against falls.

Keep the Spine in Line ▶ For the spine, back exercises are key. "For a beginner, a good thing to start off with are floor exercises or stretches in which you work at arching your back," says Dr. Bonnick. They're easy to learn and can be done anywhere with relative ease.

The next rung up the spine-protecting ladder might be back extensors. This calls for some mechanical assistance. "The back-extension machine, which is found in almost every health club, is probably the most underused machine and probably one of the most effective," says Dr. Bonnick. Dr. Bonnick believes this machine may be the most important tool in targeting the vertebrae.

Once you have mastered these exercises, you might feel confident enough to try a tougher one, the squat. "If you really want to stimulate the spine, you need an exercise that affects the whole structure," says William Kraemer, Ph.D., director of research at the Center for Sports Medicine, Pennsylvania State University. "Squats improve upon bone mass by providing adequate loading on the spine and hip." Squats are easier said than sweated. But if done slowly and carefully, they can be accomplished, and their benefits reaped.

Assist Your Wrist ▶ "Spine and hip fractures get most of the attention because they are the most devastating," says Dr. Bonnick. "But wrist fractures are extremely common and very painful." Dr. Bonnick has her patients target that area with wrist curls. "I have them do two or three sets of wrist curls, with plenty of rest in between," she says.

Rest is important with any exercise that requires a lot of gripping (this includes riding an exercise bike, for example). "Gripping for a long period of time without rest can boost blood pressure," says Dr. Bonnick. When doing wrist curls, do two or three sets with no more than eight repetitions for each set.

Get Hip to Your Hips ▶ For this major target zone, squats can also help. But to get an even better bull's-eye on the bone, Dr. Bonnick advises hip flexion and extension, and hip adduction and abduction. These exercises call for stretch bands, pulleys or tubing. Health clubs usually have pulley machines that allow you to do a number of exercises that work the hip.

Smooth Moves   17

People of all ages are dancing their arthritis pain away.

In her classic black leotard, her serene, smooth-skinned face faintly flushed from exertion and enthusiasm, Sarah Hyman, who's in her thirties, glides around the Manhattan dance studio. Watching her move with such ease, you'd never guess she's dancing for medicinal purposes—to get rid of the arthritis pain and stiffness that had once slowed her social life and almost ended her career.

Afflicted with rheumatoid arthritis in her early twenties, Sarah unsuccessfully used all the traditional weapons to battle the disease that freezes joints, weakens muscles, stifles movements and suffocates spirits. "My hands would seize up after a day's work," the physical therapist says. "I could hardly make dinner, and I couldn't go out socially because I needed to rest. I didn't want to give up full-time work and give in to my illness—I wanted to plug on, and I was sure there was a way around it."

There was a way all right: dance. Sarah began taking dance classes at the Milton Feher School of Dance and

Relaxation in New York City. Now, except during infrequent flare-ups, she's off medication. "Milton really tapped into exactly what I needed," she says. "I was able to work with less pain, do less damage to my joints and function better. Everything in my life changed." Milton Feher was way ahead of his time. He's been using his unique technique to help arthritis sufferers get the kinks out of their joints since he founded the school in 1945. "You can dance every motion in your life," he says. "Every motion you do, you can turn into a dance. It teaches you how the different parts of the body relate to each other. Everyone who wants to use his body better has to learn that."

New Steps to Relief

While experts have long advocated exercise for improving endurance, range of motion and flexibility in patients whose swollen, inflamed joints threaten to shut down completely, dance has only recently started to gain acceptance as arthritis therapy. Because cutting a rug is a cutting-edge approach to the age-old disease, dance classes especially for people with arthritis are few and far between. But you may be able to work a typical square, swing or salsa class into your therapy routine, with the advice of your doctor or physical therapist.

"Dance can increase or preserve your range of motion. It can be a strengthening exercise, because you're doing repeated motions to build muscles. And it's an endurance exercise," says Jeanne Hicks, M.D., deputy chief of rehabilitation medicine at the National Institutes of Health. "It also lifts depression, improves self-image and increases socialization."

Even more important, dancing is fun. "Many people miss the joy of moving their bodies when they get arthritis, and dancing is a great way for them to keep going," says arthritis researcher Frank R. Schmid, M.D., professor of medicine at Northwestern University.

Feher's not your typical Arthur Murray–type instructor. He's a former professional dancer who studied with the likes of Martha Graham and performed on Broadway and with international ballet companies. In his classes,

Feher uses some traditional jazz-dance moves as well as simple ballet steps to align the body. But he emphasizes relaxation, posture and body awareness—something most dance instructors don't do enough. Great emphasis is put on walking correctly, which is so important to arthritis victims. Feher himself had been felled by arthritis in his knees, cutting short his career in the early 1940s.

"I was taught to keep my legs straight by tightening my muscles," he says. "When I was studying with Martha Graham, I was so charley-horsed after class, so stiff, that it was very hard to walk up the stairs. My knees pulsed with pain."

Through study, meditation, perseverance and a certain amount of trial and error, Feher transformed the very activity that crippled him—dance—into his remedy. He says he discovered that relaxation is the key to strength, grace and better posture. "Most people don't relax naturally, so their bodies are in the wrong position and their muscles have to strain to keep them aligned," he says. "A relaxed body straightens itself." He's a testament to the success of his own technique: At 79, he still teaches five days a week and gets in a couple of tennis matches with his wife and student, Marga.

"I always thought if I kept my legs stiff, it would hold me up better," says Esther Stern, an arthritis sufferer and Feher student for more than three years. "But now, I 'ease my knees.' The pain is much less than it was, and I can walk for miles."

Feher begins and ends each hour-long class with relaxation and stretching exercises that get his students' minds on their bodies. "Most people are so busy learning the steps that they ignore the body; they don't feel the body," he says. "When you dance, you have to be aware of how your body moves and feels, not necessarily the mechanics of the steps."

Move It or Lose It

Feher's classes draw a mix: men and women, former and current dancers, opera singers, lawyers, doctors, bankers, young and not-so-young. One student, Clare

Willi, recently celebrated her 100th birthday—and almost 30 years as a Feher protégée. She completes the class, three times a week, as easily as some students half her age. Spine military-straight, Clare has none of the stooping forward, bent knees or shuffling steps that we attribute to arthritis and old age.

"Age has almost nothing to do with it," says Feher, who's featured along with other resilient septuagenarians in a new book, *Going Strong,* by Pat York. "It's understanding how the mind and body fit together. If you're not aware of your body, you allow all your bad habits to frustrate the natural motion."

Some experts believe the disease itself can't take all the blame for many of arthritis sufferers' afflictions. "So many of the problems aren't from the arthritis per se— it's the inactivity, poor posture and poor body mechanics that come from being sedentary," says Marian Minor, Ph.D., assistant professor at the University of Missouri School of Medicine. Pain—and, perhaps, medically prescribed bed rest—makes people with arthritis think they can't or shouldn't exert themselves. "We told them what not to do and created a kind of second disease."

Arthritis therapy has come a long way since doctors routinely sidelined their patients because they believed activity would make stiff joints even stiffer. "Joints often do as well, if not better, when they're used, even if they're not totally normal," Dr. Schmid says.

In one study, the late Susan G. Perlman, M.D., and Karen J. Connell and their colleagues found that a group of men and women with rheumatoid arthritis walked quicker, had less pain and swelling in their joints and experienced less depression after 16 weeks in the dance-based exercise program EDUCIZE. The group, ranging in age from 27 to 81, met for two hours twice a week. The first hour was devoted to exercise: 15 to 20 minutes of warm-up stretching and relaxation, 20 to 30 minutes of low-impact dance movements and 15 to 20 minutes of muscle-strengthening and flexibility exercises.

During the second hour, EDUCIZE participants discussed how they could use their newfound physical prowess to do things they couldn't do before, like shopping or returning to work—even little things like scrubbing the bottom shelves of the refrigerator or taking a bath.

"An arthritic person may be more hesitant," Dr. Schmid says. "They may think, 'If I do this, I'll hurt myself, or I'll end up being crippled.' " But that didn't bear out in the study. "One of the concerns the researchers had in the beginning was that damage might occur, but that didn't happen. The patients were physically better off."

If you're stepping out for the first time, your rusty joints might give you some grief. "But many of the things you'll feel, particularly if you have been inactive for a period of time, are the same things anybody would feel when they start to become more active again," says Dr. Minor.

This study didn't compare the EDUCIZE-ing participants with arthritis sufferers in traditional physical therapy programs. So it offers no scientific proof that dance is better than other therapy programs. There's also little evidence that dance specifically can delay the crippling and deformity of joints. But there is research backing range-of-motion exercise programs for flexibility and posture, as well as studies that suggest that exercise increases strength. In addition, aerobic exercise may improve endurance and function in everyday activity. Dance, which includes these forms of exercise, may also be beneficial.

Addicted to Fun

The dancers in Dr. Perlman's study seemed to approach life with more vigor than before. Many of Feher's students can also attest to that. "I've become addicted to Milton's class because I feel so much better," says Esther, who's in her late sixties. "When you finish a class, you're just raring to go. It's a lift. I'm also not a very disciplined person when it comes to exercise, so the dance class is good for me."

The physical results have a lot to do with it. "If you

161

(continued on page 164)

PUT YOUR BEST FOOT FORWARD

If you're anxious to dance your arthritis away, make sure you proceed with caution. "Dancing is better tolerated when people have minimal arthritis," says Jeanne Hicks, M.D., deputy chief of rehabilitation medicine at the National Institutes of Health. "Some people with moderate arthritis and noninflamed joints may comfortably dance. You're trying to ward off the disability of the disease, to stay in the best shape you can. However, if you have a severely involved joint, it may be too painful to dance." But that doesn't mean an arthritis veteran shouldn't give it a try—just make sure that you follow these precautions.

Get the go-ahead from your doctor. "Arthritis can affect other organ systems like the lungs and heart," Dr. Hicks says. If you have heart disease or high blood pressure, you might have to take it more slowly at the beginning and build up gradually.

Make sure you get down to specifics—explain the type of dance, how often you'll be doing it and for what period of time. Also, tell your doctor if you've had any joint replacements. If you have fluid in a large joint, like your knee, you may have to have your rheumatologist or orthopedist remove the fluid before you can comfortably begin dancing. And some people with severe rheumatoid arthritis and osteoarthritis may have loose ligaments that'll keep them off the dance floor.

Heed the Boy Scout motto: Be prepared. "One mistake people make is that they jump into these recreational programs without doing any other type of preparation," Dr. Hicks says. She suggests beginning a home program of range-of-motion, stretching and strengthening exercises about one month before your first class. Then, go through these exercises as a warm-up before each dance class and night on the town. Ask your doctor to refer you to a physical therapist who can teach you appropriate exercises.

The Arthritis Foundation has produced two videotapes with stretching, strengthening and endurance exercises. Levels one and two of the PACE (People with Arthritis Can Exercise) tapes are available from the PACE Order Center, 1800 Robert Fulton Drive, Reston, VA 22091. Or call (800) PACE-236. The price per tape is $12.50, or $24 for both.

Tell your instructor you have arthritis. Make sure he or she knows which joints are affected and when you're feeling pain.

Don't ignore a flare-up. Increased warmth, swelling and pain signal a problem. "When you have an actively inflamed joint that is red and swollen, that's not the time to vigorously exercise," says Marian Minor, Ph.D., assistant professor at the University of Missouri School of Medicine. "You need to give it extra rest and very gentle range-of-motion movement, because it's very vulnerable to damage."

Assert your wallflower power. Know when you've had enough and take a breather. "Sometimes I hurt, and I have to stop, so I'll go over and lean on the couch or sit down for a minute or two till I can go back into the class," says Esther Stern, a star student at Milton Feher's dance class in New York City. "But I'm not embarrassed. We don't try to impress each other in class."

Wear comfortable shoes. Your feet are major shock absorbers—so go low on the heels.

feel better and you're increasing your strength and endurance, you're also improving your general well-being and self-image," Dr. Hicks says. "You can do more, so you feel better about yourself."

Isolation—from being limited physically—is one of the major causes of depression among people with arthritis, experts say. Signing up for a swing class at the Y with your partner or a friend may be just what you need. "Even those of us who don't have any particular diagnostic reason may feel a little bit of apprehension—'How am I going to look? Will I be able to keep up?' But if you have a friendly person with you, maybe even with similar abilities, it's much more fun," Dr. Minor says.

But watch out—you might not be able to get enough! "Most people who exercise, whether they have arthritis or not, do it because they're having a good time," she says. "They might start for health reasons, but they continue because they enjoy it."

Looking Good

Lose Weight and Eat More

18

The trick is cutting fat, not forgoing food.

Weight-loss experts agree it's possible to lose as many as six inches in 60 days—without putting yourself through diet-and-fitness boot camp.

That is, of course, a combined total of inches from a variety of areas, including your waist, hips, thighs and other problem spots. And the slimming won't all be due to weight loss. Some of it will come from toning up flabby muscles.

Here is a simple, two-part weight-loss/shape-up plan, followed by a lot of slim-down tips and ideas that'll help make the plan fun and effective. Remember, though, it's a good idea to check with your physician before beginning a weight-loss regimen, especially if you have a medical condition or are taking medication.

Cut the Fat

Rather than having you count calories or reduce your overall food intake (as you would on most diets), this plan asks you to simply cut your fat intake. Ounce for ounce, fat contains more calories than either protein or carbohydrates, and it can end up as body fat on your hips, stomach and thighs a lot easier. Replacing fatty foods with low-fat alternatives is a much more enjoyable and much easier way to lose a few pounds than the usual crash-or-starve schemes.

The easy way to gauge an acceptable fat intake is to count grams of fat in your diet. (It's easier than counting calories.) Follow these general guidelines: If you're a woman, consume no more than 44 grams of fat per day; if you're a man, no more than 67 grams. These figures are based on people's average daily calorie intakes—around 1,600 for women, 2,400 for men. If you think your calorie intake is much lower or much higher than this, you can adjust your fat intake accordingly. For every 200 calories above or below these numbers, add or subtract 5 to 6 grams of fat.

These suggested fat limits can give you a diet in which no more than 25 percent of the calories you eat come from fat. You probably already consume more than this—most people do. (The average intake is about 40 percent of calories from fat.) So cutting down your fat to 25 percent will most likely give you a significant savings that translates into substantial weight loss—especially when combined with exercise.

It's easy to crowd some of the fatty foods out of your diet—just eat a lot of fresh vegetables and fruits. Don't confine this harvest to meals. They can be eaten as refreshing snacks throughout the day. With the exception of avocados and nuts, most plant foods won't add enough fat to your diet to be worth mentioning.

The foods that should be mentioned—and monitored for fat—are meats, dairy products and many baked goods. Beware, too, of processed foods that may have fat added, like some canned soups or frozen convenience foods. You can limit your fat intake in these food groups by making substitutions you're already familiar with: Use poultry, fish and lean red meat; low-fat (1 percent or less) milk, cheeses (five grams or less fat per one-ounce serving) and yogurt; baked goods made with a minimum of fat.

For most packaged goods, read the nutritional information on the label to find out how many grams of fat there are in a serving. Don't be fooled by a listed serving amount that's unrealistically small. Multiply that number by what you really eat.

Activate Yourself

Many people who want to lose weight aren't over-eaters; they're underexercisers. They're basically inactive. So when they do get out to exercise, they join the limping army of "weekend warriors." After going all out, these warriors are exhausted or injured, so they sit around till the next Saturday and repeat the process.

Rather than one day of perspiration followed by six of recuperation, this plan recommends spreading out your exercise over three or four days each week (each workout day followed by a less-strenuous day). Each exercise session should last a minimum of 30 minutes and a maximum of an hour. Exercise can be defined loosely as any sustained activity that will boost your heart rate above its resting pace for that period. You'll burn off much more fat with regular, moderate workouts than you would with occasional intense activity.

You also need to firm up as you lose pounds. This means including exercises that help build muscle as you burn fat, resulting in a firmer, stronger body that fits into swim wear a whole lot easier. It's known as resistance training. Even everyday chores, like digging in a flower or vegetable garden for half an hour, can have resistance-training value.

What can all these various activities do for you? Just for starters: The additional resistance training burns extra calories as it builds muscle. And muscle itself is much more metabolically active than fat tissue, so as you add muscle mass, you may increase your body's rate of burning calories during normal, everyday activities.

Of course, this is only a good estimate: The actual number of calories you'll burn varies slightly depending on your weight, fluctuations in the intensity of your workout and several other factors. But the changes all add up more quickly than you'd think, especially when combined with dietary changes.

Don't try too much too soon, though: Acclimate yourself slowly. If you haven't been very active up to now, start with something simple, like walking. For the first week: Walk at a moderate pace for 20 minutes on day one. Rest on day two. Add 10 minutes to subsequent workouts (every other day) until you are walking at a moderate pace for an hour.

Before each exercise session, do some gentle stretching exercises for about five minutes. Concentrate on the muscles you know you'll be working the hardest: legs for walking, arms for swimming and so on. After your work-

169

out, spend five minutes doing some sort of cool-down—even if you just walk around. And finally, be sure to alternate the type and intensity of your exercises to keep your self-structured program manageable and constantly interesting.

Slimming Tips

Put into regular practice, the following suggestions can help you fulfill your weight-loss/shape-up plan.

Beat the Heat ▶ During the summer months, exercising outdoors can be uncomfortable, especially in urban and suburban areas where buildings, sidewalks, rocks and roads absorb heat during peak hours, then radiate it as the air cools. Overnight, much of the absorbed heat dissipates, and everything cools down. That makes morning the best time for fitness walking, tennis and other moderately strenuous activities that usually take place on pavement. And you don't have to get out there hours before Mr. Sun is peeking over the horizon: Most areas remain relatively cool until around 9:00 A.M.

If you're not the early-bird type, you can try working out after sundown. Just make sure you do it in safe, well-lit areas. Evening exercise can be a fine way to wind down and work off the tensions of the day.

Fight Fat with Fruit ▶ The keys to a low-fat breakfast are grains and fruit, including the traditional whole-grain cereal topped with sliced bananas.

Instead of butter, jam or jelly, try one of the commercial all-fruit spreads on toast. Peaches and other fruits can be eaten whole instead of being cut up onto cereal. Berries are a good side dish.

Power Up with Protein ▶ Make sure you get some protein at breakfast—it'll give you the extra energy you need to make it through to lunch. Low-fat dairy foods are a good source of protein in the morning: skim milk on cereal, yogurt or low-fat cottage cheese with fruit. If you crave a little meat once in a while, have a slice of Canadian bacon. It's much lower in fat than regular bacon or sausages, making it an okay once-in-a-while treat.

Don't Trust Your Thirst ▶ The average person loses 2½ to 3 quarts of water per day through regular bodily functions like sweating, urinating and even breathing. And of course, water loss increases during the warm weather. Some of this loss is replaced by water in the foods we eat. But we all need to drink a minimum of eight eight-ounce glasses of water per day.

Problem is, by the time you feel thirsty, you're already low on water. It's like having a gas gauge that doesn't move off "full" until the tank goes down to three-quarters. For that reason, it's a good idea to drink eight ounces more than you think you need when you start to get thirsty. That helps you make up the fluid deficit when alerted by this not-so-early warning system.

Fight Fat and Thirst with "Waterlogged" Foods ▶ By eating more fruits and vegetables, you can maintain or even increase the amount of water you get from your diet. Naturally waterlogged snacks include watermelon, celery, nearly all types of crisp greens and most juicy fruits like grapes, peaches and plums.

Freshen Up the Fountain ▶ For a change of pace (and flavor) with your water intake, check out the many flavored mineral waters on the market. You can also flavor your own water with a little lemon or lime juice.

Make Your Own Soda ▶ Cut your favorite fruit juice by 50 percent or more with seltzer or sparkling mineral water. You'll have a refreshing, low-calorie alternative to regular soda.

Screen Out Mr. Sun ▶ When exercising outdoors during the day, it's advisable to wear sunscreen with an SPF (sun protection factor) of at least 15. You can also wear a light, breathable hat to keep the sun off your face and head. Wear a waterproof sunscreen if you'll be swimming: The sun's rays reflect off the surface of the water, increasing the skin area in danger of sunburn.

These precautions can help keep you looking as young as you feel and may even save you from skin cancer in your later years.

Hit the Ol' Swimmin' Hole ▸ Swimming is still a number-one, fun-in-the-sun (or fun-indoors) sport. It not only gives you a good aerobic workout, it has considerable resistance-training value as well. Indulge yourself with a dip any time you can.

Walk in the Water ▸ You can walk in thigh-deep water for a good leg workout. Chest-high water gives you an opportunity to exercise your arms by swinging them underwater. And you can water-walk with a buddy and carry on a conversation.

To increase the vigor of your workout in chest-deep water, you can wear an old, long-sleeved, button-down shirt. A loose piece of clothing adds to your resistance in the water.

Select the Nutritional Power Plants ▸ You should make sure you're getting plenty of nutrients from the food you eat. The following foods are especially nutrient-dense and low-fat: cauliflower, broccoli, cabbage, carrots, cantaloupe, nearly all dark green, leafy vegetables, green bell or sweet red peppers, berries and cherries.

Be a Tropical Explorer ▸ Good nutrition begins at home—but it shouldn't end there. If your supermarket stocks exotic fruits and vegetables, why not give them a try? Many tropical treats are loaded with vitamins and minerals. For example, an average cherimoya can supply more than 12 percent of your daily calcium needs and more than 15 percent of the day's iron. It also provides more than a third of the U.S. Recommended Daily Allowance (USRDA) for niacin, thiamine and riboflavin.

A papaya can provide 144 percent of the USRDA of vitamin C and more than half of your vitamin A needs through its beta-carotene content. And the guava is virtually monarch of the C suppliers—it provides as much as 275 percent of the average person's daily vitamin C needs.

Pick Your Own ▶ Combine exercise and good nutrition: In summer, go to a "pick-your-own" farm. Strawberries, peaches, peas and string beans are just a few of the crops available at pick-your-own places. And as anyone who's done it knows, all the bending, reaching, plucking, balancing and carrying is good, steady exercise. (Just try walking around with a bushel of peaches.) Check a newspaper for places near you.

Eat It Raw ▶ Hate to slave over a hot stove? Many of the vegetables you'd normally cook are delicious when eaten raw. Not just carrots but cauliflower, broccoli, string beans, peas (edible-pod varieties are especially good) and others, either plain or dipped in a light vinaigrette. You can make an entire meal out of veggie "finger foods."

Walk along the Beach ▶ Don't stroll like a beachcomber, but walk with purpose to get the maximum workout. You increase the intensity (and calorie burning) of your walking 30 to 50 percent by sand trekking.

Don't Worry about Salt Loss ▶ Perspiration contains small amounts of compounds (like salt) and minerals (like potassium) known as electrolytes. In the body they help regulate the natural electrical pulses of the heart.

These common electrolytes are important, but you won't lose dangerous amounts of them during an hour or two of moderate exercise. It's far more important to replace lost fluids than to worry about electrolytes.

A number of scientifically formulated "sports drinks" on the market advertise the importance of electrolyte replacement. There's no reason not to use them, but most of the time the average exerciser really doesn't need them. You can make your own sports drink by mixing half fruit juice and half water. Don't take salt tablets or potassium supplements to replace perspiration losses—it is unnecessary and could be dangerous.

173

Slow Down Your Appetite by Souping It Up ▶ Eating a bowl of soup before dinner can fill you up enough to curtail your food intake during the meal. Researchers at Johns Hopkins University School of Medicine served equal calorie-controlled portions of tomato soup, melon chunks or cheese and crackers to a dozen nondieting volunteers, then measured the amount of a second course (either casserole or grilled cheese sandwiches) each volunteer ate afterward. Tomato soup turned out to be the most satisfying appetizer of the three appetizers.

Other studies suggest that the warmth of the soup and its saltiness don't play major roles in making it satisfying. It just seems that soup in general has a greater effect on appetite than other common appetizers. The stomach doesn't care how many calories are in a food. A major part of what determines how satisfied we are is how much room a particular food takes up in the stomach. So a high-volume, low-calorie food like soup can satisfy us quite well.

Soup also pulls the wool over appetite-control centers in the brain: It takes a while to eat it, so it seems like you've eaten more than you actually have. The pleasant taste and texture of soup make it more satisfying on a sensory level than just plain water (or many other liquids). So slurp away!

Join an Aqua-Aerobics Program ▶ It's similar to regular aerobics, but it's done in the shallow end of a pool. It's true you won't achieve the same type of heart-pounding workout that you can during landlubber aerobics—you'll burn only about half as many calories, minute for minute, in the water. But aqua-aerobics has other benefits.

First, people who otherwise couldn't do aerobics—the elderly, the severely overweight and those who are recovering from a joint or muscle injury—are able to perform aqua-aerobics because the water supports and cushions their every move. There's a much lower risk of injury.

Second, exercising underwater is like resistance training without weights. It can gently strengthen muscles all over your body.

Many fitness clubs, YWCAs, YMCAs and even public

174

pools offer aqua-aerobics classes. Check a newspaper and call around to find a class in your area. Once you learn some of the moves, you can do them on your own any time you're at the pool.

Here are a few simple exercises you can try on your own.

■ Arm sweep: In chest-high water, put one foot in front of the other and bend your knees until your shoulders are submerged. Hold your arms straight out in front of you, palms down. Then swing your arms down past your sides and behind you as far as you can comfortably go. Turn your palms forward and swing back up. (Do 10 repetitions. Over time, work up to 20.)

■ Thigh scissors: Put your back against the pool wall in shoulder-deep water, straighten your arms out to your sides (hands at shoulder height), and grasp the ledge of the pool to support yourself. Bending at the hips with your legs straight, pull your feet and legs up until you form an L. Flex your ankles so your toes point up. Begin the exercise by moving your legs apart, then pulling them together and trying to cross them at the thighs. It helps if you keep your tummy tucked in and your lower back pressed against the pool wall. (Start with 5 repetitions. Over time, work up to 15.)

■ Figure eights: In chest-high water, put one foot in front of the other and bend your knees until your shoulders are submerged. Put your arms straight out to each side, palms down. Inscribe figure eights with your arms, keeping your fingers together. (Start with 10 repetitions. Work up to 20.)

■ Leg swings: Put your back against the pool wall in shoulder-deep water, straighten your arms to your sides, and grasp the ledge of the pool to support yourself. Bending at the hips, legs straight, pull your feet and legs up until you form an L. Flex your ankles so your toes point up, keeping your legs together. Begin the exercise by swinging both legs toward one side, then forward to the middle and back to the other side. (You don't have to touch the walls.) Contract your abdominal muscles while you swing your legs. (Start with 8 repetitions—4 to the left; 4 to the right. Work up to 16.)

19   Saving Face

Essential tips for restoring
and maintaining perfect skin.

Too little time: It's what gets in the way of creating low-fat meals from scratch and meeting your fitness goals every day without fail. When time gets tight, however, the first things that give are the nonessentials. That may include the pampering that goes into our daily skin-care regimens. Some nights, it seems, we barely have time to wash our faces.

So how do you put your best face forward, even with the busiest of schedules? This is what we asked leading dermatologists. We wanted to know what the specialists feel are the barest essentials—steps we can't afford to shortchange—for healthy, young-looking skin.

Use a Sunscreen

This was the number-one—and only unanimous—response from the dermatologists, who say smoothing on a sunscreen before you head outdoors is the most important skin-care measure you can take.

"The sun gradually destroys your skin's connective tissue, disrupting the collagen and elastic tissue and causing premature aging," explains Karen Burke, M.D., Ph.D., clinical member of Scripps Clinic and Research Foundation in La Jolla, California. "Furthermore, the outer layer of your skin thickens to protect the vital inner layers, making your skin leathery and old looking."

176
■

"Sun damage is responsible for most of what we think of as skin's aging, such as wrinkles, as well as for discoloration, growths and skin cancers," says Jeffrey H.

Binstock, M.D., assistant clinical professor of dermatologic surgery at the University of California, San Francisco.

"The bottom line is that if you're going to be outside in the sun, even for a short period of time, you should wear a sunscreen."

Moisturize

Don't wait until your skin feels dry. Moisturize regularly to prevent moisture loss. "This is especially true in winter, when the dry heat inside and the dry cold outside combine to dehydrate even the youngest skin," says Ronald Savin, M.D., clinical professor of dermatology at Yale University. He suggests that you modify your moisturizing program to suit your environment. "To combat the drying effects of winter, I recommend using a lubricant that's heavy. As the weather becomes milder and there's more humidity in the air, you can switch to a lighter lotion."

Always apply moisturizer to a freshly cleansed face, while it's still damp, to seal in the moisture. If your environment is particularly dry, mist your face with water and reapply moisturizer every few hours.

Don't forget the rest of your body, too. Keep your favorite lotion handy at the sink and at your desk for emergency hand treatment. For best results, dampen your hands first, then slather on the cream.

Remember that certain areas, such as elbows and feet, may need a heavier moisturizer than others. If you find this is true for your hands, but you don't like the stickiness of the heavier products, wait until bedtime. After your evening shower or bath, treat your dry zones to a richer moisturizer and tuck yourself between the sheets.

Now here's a timesaving tip: For daylight hours, use a moisturizer that contains sunscreen. You cut your treatment time in half.

Don't Shortcut Cleansing

Washing is the first skin-care lesson we're taught, and perhaps because it's so basic people tend not to reevaluate what they're doing. "Different skin types need different types of care, and this includes how you keep them clean," points out Dr. Binstock.

"Dry skin needs cleansing bars or lotions, while oily complexions may benefit from real soap. And everyone benefits from a gentle technique—no scrubbing or rubbing," he adds.

Gary Monheit, M.D., assistant professor of dermatology at the University of Alabama Medical School, agrees with the importance of a good cleansing routine. He also suggests:

■ If you have dry skin, cleanse once a day, in the evening. In the morning, just rinse with cool water.

■ If you have oily skin, cleanse twice a day. Use a washcloth and gently roll it over your skin to remove the dead skin layer. This mild exfoliation helps new skin underneath to grow. Without this removal, skin growth rate slows, skin begins to look sallow, and its texture becomes more wrinkled.

20 Basics in Hair Care

*Tips for keeping your
hair strong and shiny.*

Do you want your hair to set a shining example? You can ensure an attractive sheen by knowing how to use hair-care products in ways that build health and minimize damage.

Shine is directly related to the health and cleanliness of each hair's outer layer, the cuticle. Seven layers of clear cuticle cells help keep harmful chemicals from penetrating to the inner core of the hair and causing damage. The cuticle also protects against excessive evaporation of the water needed to keep your hair supple. When healthy, cuticle cells lie flat but slightly overlapping, like the shingles on a roof. When light hits them, it's reflected smoothly, creating shine. Anything that scatters the cuticle's reflection or dulls it lessens the gleam.

Unfortunately, the cuticle can be damaged by any number of everyday occurrences—excess heat, ultraviolet radiation from the sun, simple tangling and harsh chemicals. When this happens, the cells lift like shingles in a storm, and these roughed-up cuticle cells don't all reflect light in the same direction. The result is dull-looking hair.

Simple Shampoos

Dirt is the most common culprit that robs hair of its luster. The solution: choosing the right shampoo. The cleansing action of a shampoo is provided by a group of cosmetic ingredients called surfactants. They help loosen dirt, dead cells, oil and other debris so that they can be rinsed away easily .

By combining the right surfactants with other cosmetic ingredients, a basic cleansing shampoo can be developed for oily, normal or dry hair. "Start by looking for a reputable brand that states on the label that it's for your hair type," says John Corbett, Ph.D., vice-president of technology for Clairol, Inc. "But there's no single surfactant that's the best for everyone with your hair type. So you may have to try a few before you find which works best for you."

You might also want to look for a shampoo that's pH-balanced (meaning a pH between 5 and 6). A shampoo with too low a pH (below 5) won't lather as well, which is essential for removing particulate dirt, such as dust, that must be lifted from the scalp or hair before it can be rinsed out.

Hair Conditioning

But shampooing is only the first step. Conditioners contain ingredients that fill in nicks on the hair shaft and smooth the cuticle. They help hair shine by making each individual hair glisten.

They also help by cutting down the amount of static in your hair. Static keeps hairs from lying smoothly together and allows them to tangle more readily, reducing shine.

179
■

"Your hair naturally has a lot of negative ionic charges along the shaft," says Rebecca Caserio, M.D., clinical assistant professor of dermatology at the University of Pittsburgh. "This causes static. Conditioners add a positive charge, which helps neutralize the static."

"When the hairs lie together better," explains Dr. Corbett, "shine from one hair is reinforced by that of the adjacent hair. What the eye perceives as shine is actually groups of hairs lying parallel to one another to reflect the light."

Conditioners help protect hair from outside assaults and repair damage that's already done. But there is a genuine difference among the ingredients used in conditioners. If your hair is already damaged, it's especially important to understand the cause and choose a conditioner that will counteract the specific problem. For example, if your hair is very dry, look for conditioners with small amounts of oil in them. Look on the label for dimethicone or mineral oil. For fine hair, select a conditioner with a watery consistency, such as a spray-on type that you leave on.

There are two main ways to go about conditioning your hair: using a combination "conditioning shampoo" or a separate conditioner.

Conditioning shampoos, which combine the two functions in one product, work best for people whose hair is not heavily damaged. The advantage to this approach is ease. The disadvantage is that they don't clean as well as plain cleansing shampoos and don't condition as well as separate conditioners. The surfactants keep the conditioners from clinging to the hairs, and the conditioners keep the surfactants from cleaning as well as they could.

A good compromise is to alternate the two. Try using a basic cleansing shampoo for every third or fourth washing and a conditioning shampoo the rest of the time.

If your hair is fragile, damaged or dry, you probably need to use a separate conditioner. Just remember that conditioners are formulated to cling to the hair shaft and not be rinsed away. With repeated use, this film can build up and attract dirt, leaving your hair looking limp. Occasional use of a simple cleansing shampoo can keep this buildup from becoming a problem.

Preventing Hair Abuse

Even the best treatment products can't undo the daily abuse to which some of us subject our hair. You've got to abolish the root cause.

Product buildup is a common offender. It can occur as a result of continual use of any product that works by leaving a coating on the hair. And it's certainly not surprising, especially when you think of all the products people use when trying to style damaged hair. "The toughest culprits to get out are hair spray and other styling aids," says Dr. Caserio. They can leave your hair extremely dull, dry and susceptible to heat damage.

"A typical worst-case scenario is hair that's been over-permed to the point where it's frizzy," says Dr. Caserio. "Then, to get a curl, some people use hair fixatives with their curling irons or other heat-styling tools. Used together, this combination of intense heat and lacquer can actually cause the hair to be scorched."

Another big problem is holding your hair directly against the source of the heat for too long. This evaporates the water in the hair shaft that keeps it strong and pliable. The same problem arises if you blow-dry your hair past the point where it's dry to the touch. This lack of moisture makes hair so brittle it's damaged by just pulling a comb through it.

But styling instruments aren't damaging to the hair if they're used properly. (And high-quality hair appliances are designed to maintain a certain heat level that helps prevent hair scorching.) Don't hold a curling iron in one spot for more than three to five seconds.

To blow-dry for minimum damage and maximum shine:

■ Towel-dry hair before you blow-dry. It's faster and easier on your hair.

181

■ Use your blow dryer on a low setting.

- Hold it at least six inches from your head.

- Keep the dryer moving so the airflow isn't directed at the same spot for more than a few seconds.

- Gently finger-comb your hair while it's drying to prevent tangles and stress.

- Don't overdry any one section. The top layer of your hair is particularly susceptible because it's the most weathered. Stop before this area is bone-dry.

- Blow-dry the top hairs last. Make a part across the back of your head from ear to ear. Comb the upper section of hair forward and secure with clips. Start drying at the nape of the neck and work upward toward the crown. When you've dried that section, bring another layer of hair down. Continue working toward the front. Finish with the sides.

Waves and Hues

Permanent waves and hair coloring are double-edged swords. It's true that any chemical treatment can damage hair, but if done right, perms and color are terrific boosters for lackluster locks. In uncolored hair, the cuticle is flat and reflects light from the top layer. If the hair is damaged, light penetrates more deeply—perhaps all the way to the innermost layer of cuticle cells. When it's finally reflected, the light bounces around willy-nilly between the layers, reducing the cohesive surface reflection that makes hair glisten. Hair coloring can help because it's absorbed by the cuticle and causes the cuticle to give a smoother reflection.

If your hair is already damaged, though, you're probably better off with semipermanent hair coloring—it adds color without the damage of the so-called permanent colors because it doesn't roughen the surface of the cuticle.

And if your hair really does look better with a perm, just set your mind on keeping damage to a minimum. "Everybody gets a little breakage after a perm," says Dr. Caserio. "That's normal and really doesn't show." Perms become harmful when you have them too often or too soon after a coloring treatment. Generally you should wait 12 weeks between perms. And don't color and perm hair at the same time—perm first and wait one to two weeks to color. Avoid these mistakes and your hair should keep its radiant glow.

Shine Those Pearly Whites

21

Strategies for having whiter, brighter teeth.

Not everyone is fortunate enough to be born with a 1,000-watt smile. But most people can brighten and whiten their teeth with simple, home-based strategies— or with a little help from a dentist.

Knowing the cause of the discoloration may help you find the right cure. Stained, streaked or darkened teeth can be caused by the following factors.

Food Prints ▶ Coffee, tea, wine, grape juice and acidic soft drinks can cause minor surface stains.

The Passing of Time ▶ Sure, your hair grays as you age, but so does the color of your teeth. Years of wear and tear cause minor cracks in the enamel. They can darken its appearance and attract stains.

Medication That Mars ▶ The antibiotic tetracycline can sometimes stain teeth if taken early—from birth up to about eight years.

Too Much of a Good Thing ▶ If you grew up in a community that had too much natural fluoride in the water, your teeth may be stained with white speckles or brown pigment.

Accidents and Other Mishaps ▶ Injury to a tooth can cause staining. So can early childhood illness, such as a lengthy, severe fever, scarlet fever or severe jaundice. And some inherent tooth disorders, such as congenitally malformed teeth, can roughen the surface, causing teeth to darken.

Looking on the Bright Side

Returning your teeth to their former color can be as simple as starting with the basics.

Wield Your Toothbrush ▶ Food stains can be held in check—even prevented—if you brush thoroughly and often. Plaque, the bacteria-laden film that forms on teeth, has an insidiously sticky way of grabbing hold of other residues, making teeth look darker. If it's left undisturbed for too long, plaque turns into yellow tartar.

Eye Your Diet ▶ If you find yourself partaking of a suspected tooth darkener (like coffee or tea) in large quantities, ease off and see if there's any improvement.

Take Your Teeth to the Cleaners ▶ A lot of tooth discoloration—particularly food or tobacco—can be erased by a thorough cleaning at the dentist.

This kind of oral hygiene can also help invigorate your gums. Red, puffy, irritated gums tend to make teeth look darker. Bright, tight gum tissue reflects well on the teeth, making them appear brighter. Maintain your gums with regular brushing and flossing.

Consider Hitting the Bleach ▶ If none of the above are effective in subduing your stains, you might want to try bleaching. There are quite a few over-the-counter tooth-whitening products available. They come in the form of pastes or polishes—all containing weak concentrations of bleaching agents.

There's not much hard evidence out there on how well these products work. Some patients report favorable, though unpredictable, results with mild stains. "Little research exists on the long-term safety of these products, but as yet, few problems have been reported," says Joel M. Boriskin, D.D.S., chief of the Division of Dentistry at Highland General Hospital in Oakland, California. The best bet is to ask your dentist what he or she recommends.

If your discoloration is more extensive or you're more serious about kissing tooth stains goodbye, you may instead opt for in-office bleaching by your dentist or a dentist-supervised, patient-administered bleach. "These may be more expensive, but you'll benefit from the supervision and knowledge of the dentist," says Bruce Crispin, D.D.S., director of the Center for Esthetic Dentistry at UCLA.

These procedures usually employ higher concentrations of the bleaching agents found in over-the-counter products: carbamide peroxide or hydrogen peroxide. A whitening plan may include three or more treatments, and follow-up visits at one- to three-year intervals to bolster the brightness. Cost: $175 to $275 per visit.

For the dentist-supervised, patient-administered bleaching program, the dentist will make a mouth guard that is worn overnight to hold the solution against your teeth. The amount of use is controlled by the patient. If you have adverse symptoms, such as discomfort, you may not wear it often. If you don't have adverse symptoms, you can wear it several hours a day plus overnight. But if your teeth become too sensitive and it's too painful, you may have to discontinue wearing the mouthpiece.

Usually, if the patient uses it fairly regularly, they'll see results within one week. Then after three to five weeks most of the results have taken place. Cost: $175 to $350 per arch.

Most people get both the top teeth (top arch) and bottom arch done. (If someone wants to get just one or two teeth bleached, he will probably go for the dentist-administered process.)

Bond with Your Dentist ▶ If bleaching doesn't do the trick or isn't appropriate in your case, the next step is composite bonding. In this procedure, your teeth are covered with a pastelike bonding material that's hardened with high-intensity light. It lasts from three to eight years. Cost: $200 to $500 per tooth.

Put Up a Good Veneer ▶ Think of it as a press-on fingernail for your tooth. Though more expensive than composite bonding, porcelain laminates (veneers) probably last longer—10 to 12 years. The front of the tooth is painted with adhesive, then the veneer is pressed into place. Cost: $275 to $850 per tooth.

Don a Crown ▶ These jackets for the teeth may be the only option for severe stains. Crowns require more work and are more expensive than veneers. They last 10 to 12 years. Cost: $445 to $1,000 per tooth.

Beating Disease

Heart Health for Women

22

Techniques that protect the men will work for you, too.

If there's a man in your life, chances are you've given a lot of thought to protecting his heart. You help him follow a low-fat diet and encourage him to walk every day. Perhaps you even remind him to take the aspirin his physician prescribed to reduce his chance of heart attack.

But have you thought about your heart lately?

Fact is, cardiovascular disease, including heart attack and stroke, takes the life of more women than any other illness. In fact, about 247,000 of the more than 520,000 people who die from heart attack each year are women. (By comparison, about 40,500 women die each year from breast cancer.)

"Heart disease is only now being recognized for the silent epidemic among women that it really is," says heart expert Dean Ornish, M.D., director of the Preventive Medicine Research Institute in Sausalito, California.

The main difference between the genders is that women get heart disease about 10 to 15 years later than men. The reason for the delay, scientists believe, is that the female hormone estrogen, produced abundantly before menopause, protects women's hearts.

What Every Woman Should Know

We know a great deal about ways to prevent men's heart disease. The vast majority of experimental trials (in which people are given preventive measures and treatments, and the results assessed) have been conducted among men, notes Millicent Higgins, M.D., of the National Heart, Lung and Blood Institute.

Only a few studies over the years have involved large numbers of women. Two of the most important: the Framingham Heart Study, in Massachusetts, which has followed about 5,000 men and women for over 40 years; and the Harvard Nurse's Health Study, which has tracked more than 121,000 female nurses for 15 years.

Assessing Your Risks

Based on those studies—and the advice of leading cardiologists—here's what you should know about assessing your risks and developing a personal protection plan (with the help of a qualified physician, of course).

Are You Past Menopause? ▶ Heart attacks rarely strike young women. Researchers believe it's because the hormones circulated before menopause—particularly estrogen—confer a special protection on young women. Estrogen raises levels of HDL (high-density lipoprotein), the "good" cholesterol, and lowers LDL (low-density lipoprotein), the "bad" kind, while a woman is young.

But between 45 and 55, the picture starts to change. Nearly all the cardiovascular disease risk factors, such as blood pressure, HDL cholesterol and LDL cholesterol, and others, move in less favorable directions as menopause approaches. By the way, there may also be an increased risk if the menopause was created "surgically." Some, but not all, of the evidence suggests a higher heart disease risk for young women whose ovaries are removed.

Do You Smoke or Spend a Lot of Time around Someone Who Does? ▶ "Smoking accounts for more than 50 percent of heart attacks in premenopausal women," says Harvard Medical School researcher JoAnn Manson, M.D.

What's more, female smokers who use oral contraceptives face double jeopardy. They're up to 39 times more likely to have a heart attack and up to 22 times more likely to suffer a stroke than women who neither smoke nor use birth control pills. Remember that "passive smoking" can be a danger. Exposure to other people's smoke may be just as bad for your heart as you yourself smoking, doctors tell us.

Do You Have High Blood Pressure? ▸ High blood pressure, for both men and women, is defined as a blood pressure reading of 140/90 or greater on several successive occasions.

Over a quarter of women from 18 to 74 have high blood pressure, and more than half of all postmenopausal women have the disease. In fact, women over 65 are more likely to develop high blood pressure than men. Black women, overweight women and women with a family history of high blood pressure are especially susceptible. Ideally, the systolic pressure (the first number of your blood pressure score) should be below 120, and the second number, the diastolic, should be below 80.

You can help reduce blood pressure by exercising, losing excess body fat, relaxing and avoiding salt. Medication is prescribed in severe cases.

Do You Have Adult-Onset Diabetes or a Strong Family History of the Disease? ▸ Adult-onset diabetes increases heart attack risk for both men and women, but more so for women. Peter Wilson, M.D., director of laboratories for the Framingham study, notes a woman diabetic has three times as great a risk of heart disease as a nondiabetic woman; a male diabetic has twice the risk of heart disease as a nondiabetic male.

Diabetes even seems to "undo" younger women's premenopausal protection. "If a woman becomes diabetic, she just became a man, in terms of heart disease risk," says Dr. Wilson.

"Any woman with a strong family history of adult-onset diabetes should be especially vigilant about eating a low-fat (heart-healthy) diet, exercising and taking steps to reduce excess weight," says David Alexander Leaf, M.D., director of the Healthy Hearts Program at the UCLA School of Medicine. "Adult-onset diabetes is a genetic tendency that can be triggered by poor health habits, especially those that lead to overweight."

Do You Have Elevated Blood Cholesterol (above 200)? ▸ We all know that high blood cholesterol levels are a major risk factor for heart disease. So far, the gen-

191

eral recommendations for women are the same as for men: To prevent increased risk of heart disease, aim to keep cholesterol at or below 200 mg/dl.

The most effective way to do that is to eat a diet low in fat, especially saturated fat. Saturated fat intake raises your blood cholesterol. Your best bet for fighting fat is to follow the American Heart Association guidelines, which aim at fewer than 30 percent of calories from fat.

Others have suggested even lower levels. Dr. Ornish puts people with evidence of heart disease on diets deriving less than 10 percent of their calories from fat. Dr. Ornish notes intriguing evidence from his research, however: While men needed to reduce their fat levels to under 10 percent of calories to reverse heart disease, he says, women who ate a slightly higher-fat diet (under 30 percent of calories from fat) showed evidence of heart disease reversal. "It's just speculation at this point, but women may be able to eat a slightly higher-fat diet than men and still reverse arteriosclerosis," says Dr. Ornish.

A low-fat diet should be initiated by women of all ages, regardless of whether they have other risk factors for heart disease.

Also, low-fat diets not only reduce cardiovascular disease risk but also may reduce risk of cancers, particularly colon cancer, the leading cause of cancer death in non-smokers. "Heart disease and colon cancer together certainly add up to a good reason for eating a low-fat diet," says Graham Colditz, M.D., an assistant professor at Harvard Medical School.

Do You Have Low HDL Cholesterol (below 55)? ▶
HDL (high-density lipoprotein) cholesterol is another marker doctors use to evaluate heart disease risk. In fact, some say it's a more accurate predictor of heart health than total cholesterol. HDLs are considered the good guys. They usher cholesterol out of the bloodstream. So the higher the HDL level in your blood, the greater your protection against heart disease. And for women, it's possible that the ideal HDL should be slightly higher than a man's.

"On average, women's HDL is about 55 mg/dl. Men

average about 45 mg/dl. Our data showed that if a woman's HDL were 45, the male average, she'd be at a much greater risk for heart disease," says Dr. Wilson. "An HDL of 55 is good for women—and higher is better."

Do You Have High Triglycerides (over 250)? ▶ Triglycerides are the chemical form in which most fats exist in the body and blood.

"In the Framingham study, we have overwhelming evidence that higher triglyceride levels are directly linked to a higher risk of heart attack in women—more so than in men," says Dr. Wilson. Currently, for both men and women, triglyceride levels from 85 to 250 mg/dl are considered normal; from 250 to 500 mg/dl are labeled "borderline high."

Are You 15 Pounds or More Overweight on Standard Weight/Height Tables? ▶ And how is that weight distributed? Are you shaped more like an apple than a pear?

"Both overweight and distribution of body weight have been correlated to heart disease risk in women," Dr. Wilson says. The Nurse's Health Study, for example, indicates an increase in risk even with mild overweight (as measured on the insurance charts). But some scientists question whether a few excess pounds on older women pose as much risk as they would on younger women. Sylvia Wassertheil-Smoller, Ph.D., professor of epidemiology at Albert Einstein College of Medicine, believes more research is needed on older women's health.

In the meantime, most physicians agree that it's prudent to maintain your weight within a reasonable range—no more than 15 pounds above your ideal weight. "The clear implications are that we could all lose some weight and be better off in terms of cardiovascular risk. For many middle-aged and older women, taking 10 to 20 pounds off is a reasonable aim," says Nurse's Health Study researcher Dr. Colditz.

Other studies have shown a greater risk in being shaped like an apple than like a pear. "When a woman

193
∎

walks into my office with a big abdomen and thin arms and legs, I worry more about her than a woman of the same weight who has a waistline but big hips and buttocks," says Marianne Legato, M.D., a cardiac researcher on the faculty of the Columbia University College of Physicians and Surgeons.

Are You Active? ▶ We know that regular aerobic exercise (such as a brisk 30-minute walk three days a week) is linked to lower total cholesterol and triglycerides, higher HDL cholesterol, lower blood pressure and weight loss. That's been well documented, mostly in men. Now researchers Jane Owens, Dr.P.H., and Karen Matthews, Ph.D., at the University of Pittsburgh, have looked at the relationship of exercise to heart disease risk factors in women. "We've shown in our studies that women who are active have lower levels of the risk factors that contribute to coronary disease, like lower blood pressure, lower total cholesterol and higher HDL cholesterol," says Dr. Owens. She adds that she and Dr. Matthews have collected data, not yet published, that suggest that women who increase their physical activity may be protected against the increasing weight and decreasing levels of HDL cholesterol (both associated with menopause).

Doctors agree, all women—regardless of age or existing risk factors—stand to benefit from regular exercise. (But first, have a physical exam.)

Do You Have a Family History of Heart Disease? ▶ Regardless of your gender, if either parent died of or developed heart disease before age 60, you have an increased risk of developing it, too. The younger their age, the greater your risk at a younger age.

Do You Currently Take Oral Contraceptives, and Are You over Age 35? ▶ Use of oral contraceptives significantly increases heart disease in women who smoke cigarettes. Do they increase the heart disease risk in non-smokers? Most studies say yes, particularly in women over age 35. But when these studies were done, birth control pills contained about twice the dose of estrogen of the newer low-dose pills. So today the risk may not be as great as it once was.

Nevertheless, the American Heart Association suggests that women over 35 choose a different form of birth control. Dr. Legato is cautious about using oral contraceptives even in younger women if they have many heart disease risk factors. (Incidentally, past use of the oral contraceptives doesn't seem to increase risk.)

Planning Your Defense

Now that you've identified your risks, you and your physician can do a better job planning your defense. Besides the specific risk-reducing measures described above, consider the following two heart-protective actions that carry multiple benefits. They're both designed to protect women who fit a certain risk profile.

Consider Taking Aspirin as a Preventive Measure ▶ Studies have shown that taking aspirin regularly can reduce the likelihood of heart attack in men. Now there's new evidence looking specifically at the impact of aspirin on women. In the first large-scale, detailed study of aspirin's ability to protect women against a first heart attack, the Nurse's Health Study found a substantial reduction in heart risk among women who use small amounts of the drug. The research was presented to the American Heart Association conference in March 1991.

The women in the study were surveyed to find out how frequently they took aspirin. Twenty-six percent of the nurses (about 23,000) reported taking at least one aspirin a week, usually for headaches or other minor pains.

"We found about a 30 percent reduction in the risk of first heart attack among women who took one to six aspirin tablets per week," says Dr. Manson, who was the lead researcher.

Dr. Manson explains that the aspirin was most beneficial for women over 50 and for women with other cardiovascular risk factors, like diabetes, smoking or high blood pressure.

Aspirin isn't for every woman, Dr. Manson adds. For premenopausal women, she says, there is no evidence that regular aspirin use is helpful in preventing heart attacks.

"It's more likely to be helpful for postmenopausal women with other cardiovascular risk factors," she adds. "And then it should be taken only under a physician's supervision."

Dr. Manson says that her study is not the final word. A trial experiment should be conducted, she says, in which women take the drug regularly and are followed up. Since the nurses took aspirin sporadically, it's even possible that the real benefit would be greater than 30 percent if women used aspirin regularly, Dr. Manson speculates.

If You Are Postmenopausal, Consider Hormone Replacement Therapy ▸ Hormone replacement therapy is typically initiated to ease hot flashes and other symptoms of menopause. But many doctors feel that the benefits go beyond that. Estrogen, they say, can save women's lives.

A recent study from the University of Southern California, for example, suggests that women who take estrogen can add up to three years to their lives, mostly because of the dramatic reduction in risk from heart disease and stroke.

Other studies support the heart-healthy effect of estrogen. For example, researchers Elizabeth Barrett-Connor, M.D., and Trudy Bush, Ph.D., reviewed 21 studies on women taking estrogen. The majority of studies (16) show a reduction in heart disease risk for women taking oral estrogen. On average, the women were 50 percent less likely to suffer a heart attack. The evidence of protection against heart disease, the authors conclude, is "strong, reasonably consistent and biologically plausible."

Exactly how estrogen does this is not completely understood. Scientists suspect that it has a favorable effect on blood pressure and increases HDL cholesterol levels. Some research indicates that estrogen protects blood vessel walls from the changes that cause fatty plaque to accumulate and may even affect heart tissue directly.

But before you go rushing off for a prescription, you should be aware that questions persist. For one thing, long-term estrogen use has been associated with uterine cancer. To protect against this, low-dose estrogen is usually given in combination with progestin, another female hormone. But we don't know whether progestin may undo some of estrogen's heart benefits.

"The concern is that, while estrogen moves lipid profiles in a positive direction, progestins may push it in a bad direction," explains Charles Hammond, M.D., chairman of the department of obstetrics and gynecology at Duke University Medical Center.

Another question that looms involves the estrogen/breast cancer connection. Estrogen replacement therapy does not cause breast cancer. But because some breast cancers are estrogen-dependent, the concern is that if a woman with an existing, undetected breast cancer takes estrogen, cancer growth could be encouraged. How much of a risk this poses is not clear—the evidence to date remains completely contradictory. Hopefully, we'll know more in a few years, as results from several major National Institutes of Health studies become available.

One study, the experimental PEPI (Postmenopausal Estrogen/Progestin Interventions) study, will examine the effects of estrogen alone, and estrogen plus progestin, on heart disease risk factors (and other conditions) in several hundred women.

In the meantime, what's a woman to do? Most researchers believe that heart protection will prove to be an overwhelming reason for most women to take estrogen after menopause. After all, heart disease is by far the biggest threat to women's lives.

However, doctors agree that the decision must be made on an individual basis, considering each woman's risk factors. Most doctors say they would not prescribe estrogen to a woman with a personal history of breast cancer. Some doctors are also reluctant to prescribe estrogen to women who have a family history of breast cancer

197
∎

or a personal history of benign breast disease.

"Clearly there are many other ways a woman can reduce her risk of heart attack, besides estrogen. She can stop smoking, maintain ideal weight and exercise," says Dr. Colditz. "As long as her blood pressure is normal and her cholesterol numbers are good, there's little reason for her to go on hormone replacement specifically for heart disease prevention." If, however, a woman has a very strong family history of heart disease and other risk factors that cannot be controlled through other means, estrogen replacement may offer some protection.

"I think it's prudent to advise women to take this therapy, particularly if they have underlying family or personal risk factors for heart disease," says Ezra Davidson, M.D., immediate past president of the American College of Obstetricians and Gynecologists. "To me, the benefits of estrogen seem overwhelming, and the breast cancer risk, though it has to be respected, is small."

Says Meir Stampfer, M.D., Dr.P.H., a leading researcher on the Nurse's Health Study who's on the faculty of Harvard Medical School, "I think every woman ought to consider hormone replacement therapy. Not every woman ought to be on it, but for most women the benefits outweigh the risks."

If you do consider this therapy, remember: Estrogens taken orally are more effective in reducing cardiovascular risks than those taken in creams or skin patches. Also, different forms of progesterone exert different effects. "The lowest-dose, most natural progesterones may be better for the heart," says Jay Sullivan, M.D., chief of the Division of Cardiovascular Diseases at the University of Tennessee.

How to Talk to Your Doctor about Your Heart

Not all physicians give much thought to women's risk of heart disease, particularly younger women's risk. "Many physicians don't even entertain the diagnosis of heart disease. They don't believe it's a significant event in the lives of women until they are very old," contends Dr. Legato, author of *The Female Heart.*

"Doctors need to be more sensitive to the risk factors," says Dr. Legato. "I have a 27-year-old woman in my practice who's the daughter of a man who had his first heart attack at 36. She smokes, she has high cholesterol, and she's been on oral contraceptives for a long time. I spoke to her gynecologist yesterday about switching her to another form of contraception. He thinks my concerns about coronary artery disease are ridiculous. They're not ridiculous!"

There are ways to get the checkups and care you need. One good start, says Dr. Legato, is to see an internist or general practitioner, if you don't already do so. "Many women depend on their gynecologists for their primary care. But gynecologists are simply not geared up to provide a complete internal assessment," she says.

Get a thorough physical, says Dr. Legato. This should include a blood pressure check and a complete lipid profile that will reveal HDL, LDL and triglycerides, along with total cholesterol levels. In addition, you should be tested for diabetes.

Don't be afraid to ask for specifics, says Dr. Wassertheil-Smoller. "Sometimes doctors say your pressure is a little high or your cholesterol is a little high. That's not enough." You need to know how high and what he or she recommends that you do about it. Use this opportunity with the doctor to discuss other risk factors you may have.

Premenopausal women should see their doctor every other year for a checkup if they're in very good health and don't have any risk factors for heart disease. If they do have risk factors, such as a family history of cardiovascular disease or diabetes, smoking or excess stress, annual checkups would be wiser, says Dr. Legato.

Menopausal women should have an annual checkup, most doctors agree, regardless of their other risk factors. Together, a woman and her physician can tackle tougher questions, like whether to undergo hormone replacement therapy.

All of this requires a caring physician, Dr. Legato notes. "It takes patience on both sides, to give and to listen to advice." But she adds, the results are worth it. "Good health is the result of a real collaboration between doctor and patient."

23 Take the "Ring" Out of Hearing

Now you can subdue the annoying sounds of tinnitus.

Rosalie Coponi first noticed the low hum in her ears about three years ago, right after a bout with the flu. At first, it wasn't much louder than the background sound of the central heater in her Allentown, Pennsylvania, home. Although she couldn't seem to shake it, she wasn't going to whine about what probably was no more than a minor annoyance. Things could be worse! And pretty soon, they were.

"The hum soon became a roar, like there was a motor running in my ear," Rosalie says. "It was so loud I couldn't think and had trouble sleeping at night. I also lost my appetite—every time I got on the scale, I weighed five pounds less. A lot of people say their ears ring sometimes—I'd had that before, too, but it was nothing like this."

Sapped of energy and unable to muster enough concentration to read, cook or clean, Rosalie went to the first of the five ear, nose and throat (ENT) specialists she was to see over the following two years of frustration and pain. There, she found a name for her affliction—tinnitus (pronounced *TIN-nih-tus* or *tin-NEYE-tus*). What she didn't find was immediate relief.

The problem with tinnitus is that it isn't a disease. It's a symptom that can be caused by any number of physical problems. In fact, anything that can go wrong with the sense of hearing can have tinnitus as a symptom. The fact that the list of possible suspects is so long makes it difficult for doctors to pinpoint the actual culprit. And it could be that more than one ailment is contributing to the problem. So curing a case of tinnitus is something of a medical mystery. But diagnosing it doesn't always have to be.

In Rosalie's case, part of the mystery was eventually solved. After a year of learning to handle stress and protecting her ears from noise, she's almost back to 100 percent. "I used to hear the noise all the time, but now I have normal days," she says. "And when I do hear it, it's lower than the original hum I started out with."

Managing the problem ends up being the goal in most instances of severe tinnitus, because while the sound source may be identified, the chances of completely correcting tinnitus are relatively slim. But even when doctors can't figure out why the volume gets cranked up on your internal sound machine, the unbearable roar can be reduced to a barely heard whisper, if not turned off altogether. And specialists at tinnitus clinics all over the world are constantly working on new ways to make diagnosis and treatment less of a gamble and more of a calculated wager.

Searching for the Secret to Your Distress

Approximately 40 to 50 million Americans experience the internal cacophony of hums, roars, buzzes or clicks that characterizes tinnitus. But for most of them, the sounds are barely noticeable, lasting anywhere from a matter of minutes to a couple of days.

Twelve million of these cases, however, are like Rosalie's. The steamy hiss, the oceanic roar, the answering-machine beep of their tinnitus drowns out most external sounds, disrupts their lives and sends them on an often lengthy, frustrating search for treatment. "If you're walking through a busy airport, for example, and you can still hear your tinnitus despite all the racket, it's probably interfering with your life—and that's when you should see a doctor," says Jack Vernon, Ph.D., professor of otolaryngology at the Oregon Hearing Research Center at Oregon Health Sciences University.

That's because, in rare cases, your ears could be signaling the presence of a tumor, a serious problem with your autoimmune system, Ménière's disease or a partially blocked artery in your neck. Those are the first problems an ear, nose and throat doctor will look for. He'll also be able to tell if you have an infection, excess fluid in your middle ear or another ear problem known to be related to tinnitus. These are clear-cut cases, and standard methods, such as surgery and drugs, can be used to treat them. In these situations there is a chance that the noise can be silenced for good.

But when there's no obvious physical reason for your ears to roar like the final lap of the Indianapolis 500, where do you go from there? "After your doctor finds that there's nothing wrong, everybody looks at you like you're crazy," Rosalie says. "But even though no one else can hear it, the problem is real, and it's devastating."

The next step is to find out if you have one or more of the other medical conditions that may cause or aggravate tinnitus. A possible culprit is the irritation and congestion caused by allergies. "With proper treatment of the allergies, you may be able to at least control your level of tinnitus or eliminate it entirely," says Ronald G. Amedee, M.D., assistant professor of otolaryngology–head and neck surgery at Tulane Medical Center. Indeed, Rosalie's roar grew much less severe once she began monthly shots for ragweed, mold and pollen allergies and stopped eating the dairy products she was allergic to.

Blood circulation problems may also be related to your tinnitus. "People who have increased blood flow to the ear due to high blood pressure may hear a sound like a heartbeat," says John House, M.D., associate clinical professor of otolaryngology at the University of Southern California School of Medicine and president of the House Ear Institute. Addressing that problem with conventional treatments, such as a low-salt diet and antihypertensive medications, may give you some welcome relief.

If you experience a pulsing tinnitus, see a cardiologist to determine the source of the pulsing. (Be aware, though, that some blood pressure medications may aggravate or cause tinnitus. Alert your regular doctor to your tinnitus should he prescribe antihypertensive drugs.) If you suspect that a medication is causing tinnitus, see your doctor.

On the flip side, if you have high blood cholesterol levels or heart disease, you may not be getting enough blood to your ear. The resulting irritation to your inner ear could be a source of tinnitus. So reducing your cholesterol level may be one way for you to combat tinnitus. In rare cases, people with tinnitus also have temporomandibular joint disorder (TMD) or bruxism (teeth-grinding disorder)—two conditions that can further aggravate an already bad problem. In those instances, prescription muscle relaxers may help.

But it's more likely that severe tinnitus is the product of direct damage to the hair cells in the ear—damage that can't be repaired. In some cases this kind of damage is the immediate result of sudden exposure to loud noises—like the hunting enthusiast who fires his shotgun one too many times, or the stationary cyclist who cranks up her personal radio a little too loud during a long ride. In other cases, the damage accumulates slowly over the years from a daily barrage of external noises—in fact, some estimates say most tinnitus sufferers are between the ages of 55 and 74.

Some antibiotics and anticancer drugs can cause tinnitus, but most don't. Other drugs that can cause or aggravate tinnitus include antidepressants, blood pressure medications and nonsteroidal anti-inflammatory drugs.

"Noise and certain drugs can damage the cells in the ear that transform sounds into the nerve impulses that travel to the brain," says Pawel J. Jastreboff, Ph.D., professor of surgery and physiology and director of the tinnitus clinic at the University of Maryland. "When someone has tinnitus, we think something is wrong with the way the nerves work in the auditory pathways of the brain. In some cases, there is an amplification that results in the 'feedback' phenomenon, which sounds similar to someone turning up the volume of a microphone too high."

Learning to Live with Tinnitus

Even though this kind of damage is irreparable, there's no need to give up. A tinnitus expert will put you through a lengthy interview and a battery of tests to get a better handle on the scope of it. Some of these tests may already be familiar to you if you've been to an ear, nose and throat doctor. But in addition to looking for hearing loss and equilibrium problems, a tinnitus expert also checks for nerve damage by analyzing the way electrical sound impulses are traveling to the brain.

And tinnitus experts also use a test that actually allows them to identify the sound of your tinnitus. With the help of a specially trained audiologist and a sound generator, a series of tones, buzzes, hisses and roars are played until they hit upon a sound that you recognize as your own. Then the loudness is also adjusted until the audiologist hears nearly the sound that you do. Tinnitus experts use all this information to determine the best approach to your problem, based on the experiences of other patients with similar profiles.

They also try to assess how you're coping with it emotionally, because that may be making it worse. "The incidence of severe stress, anxiety and depression is very high among people who have disabling tinnitus," says Abraham Shulman, M.D., professor of otolaryngology at the State University of New York at Brooklyn. "We have to give equal attention to both management of the sound and your response." So it often happens that the best way of managing tinnitus is to attack it on a number of fronts. Here are some weapons you can use to control tinnitus.

204

Ear Protection ▶ It's most important to protect your ears from loud noises, because they can make your tinnitus even worse. "I carry soft foam earplugs in my cosmetic bag and use them whenever I'm in a noisy place, because it could trigger an attack," Rosalie says. (Earplugs are available in drugstores for about $2.)

Even though most patients with severe tinnitus are over age 55, more and more young people—even teenagers—are going to see tinnitus specialists. Many experts blame blaring car and personal stereos, but sounds from snowmobiles, lawn mowers, chain saws and other equipment can also damage hearing.

Most personal and car stereos have volume-control dials that go from 1 to 10. If you currently suffer from tinnitus, a good all-around rule is to keep the volume set at 4 or below. If you don't have tinnitus and want to make sure you never get it, the same rule applies.

Avoid Ear-Damaging Substances ▶ Of course, a tinnitus specialist should take you off any drugs that are known to be ototoxic—poisonous to the ear—like the antibiotic streptomycin. But even aspirin and aspirin-containing remedies, while they don't cause permanent damage to the ear, can also induce temporary tinnitus and aggravate a permanent case when taken in moderate and, more commonly, high doses. So if you need a painkiller, try acetaminophen, or ask your doctor if ibuprofen is appropriate to take. Also, stay away from quinine and nicotine. Although experts don't know why, they seem to make the ringing worse. Alcohol and caffeine can also affect tinnitus, depending on the person. Tell your doctor how much of these you consume to see whether they are a problem.

Hearing Aids ▶ "About 95 percent of patients with tinnitus have some degree of hearing loss," says Dr. House. "Wearing a hearing aid can't get rid of the ringing, but the tinnitus may become less obvious if you can hear better." And even if you don't have a noticeable hearing loss, a hearing aid might help. Often, tinnitus sufferers have high-frequency hearing damage. While high-frequency sound waves are not crucial for speech perception, we normally hear them. When a person has

205

hearing loss, the brain is not receiving this information. So a specialist may attempt to make those sound waves available to the brain by the use of a hearing aid, even though the patient has normal hearing in the lower frequencies.

Maskers and Tinnitus Devices ▶ "My greatest joy used to be reading in a quiet room, but now that's impossible," Rosalie says. "So now I play the radio, softly, in the background, and my ears are clear. I also have a television going when I'm in the kitchen, so I can do my cooking and sewing in peace, and a radio with earphones by my bed, in case I wake up during the night and hear that hum."

That's Rosalie's way of masking—substituting another sound for the sound of her tinnitus. There actually are special masking devices—hearing-aid-like pieces that fit inside or behind the ear and emit a noise like the sound of the tinnitus into your ear. How can more noise help? "Maskers attempt to cover up the tinnitus with a lower-pitched external sound that's more acceptable and easier to ignore than the high-pitched internal sound," Dr. Vernon says.

One of the standard tests used by experts helps predict whether a masker can work for you. The patient hears a series of tones, but this time the goal is to find a sound that comfortably hides the tinnitus. If one is identified, a masking device is adjusted to mimic that soothing sound's tone and loudness.

You may not need to use the masker all the time. Your tinnitus may be temporarily unnoticeable, even after the masker is removed. Many people who have hearing loss but have had little luck with a hearing aid alone find relief with a combination hearing aid and masker, known as a tinnitus instrument.

Another approach, advocated by Dr. Jastreboff, is to not try to mask the whole range of tinnitus sounds but to introduce a stable background sound (or "white noise") that makes it easier for the brain to ignore the tinnitus. This is generally accepted in Britain but is considered new and controversial in this country.

Emotional-Relief Techniques ▶ Tinnitus sufferers are often told they need to "learn to live with it" but are seldom told how. And the frustration of dealing with a symptom that is, after all, all in your head often compounds the problem. "It's rare that treating stress or depression alone totally gets rid of tinnitus, but it's part of the whole approach, and for some people, it needs to be taken care of for treatment to be successful," Dr. Jastreboff says. "We try to teach your brain to ignore the tinnitus, to push it aside, because we can't stop the sound altogether."

The trick is finding the way of dealing with the stress or depression that's most effective for you. It may be something as simple as exercise. "Walking helps me relax, but I can't walk too fast, because it makes my ears beat," Rosalie says. "So I walk at a normal pace, and that helps me get rid of my stress."

She also found that keeping her emotions bottled up added to her stress and made her tinnitus worse. "Now I have to talk right away about anything that upsets or disturbs me, rather than keeping it in and brooding about it," she says.

Some people find relief through progressive relaxation, a technique in which the patient tenses and then relaxes different parts of his body. "I've learned to relax on my recliner so that every muscle in my body goes limp," says Morris Rubinoff, a tinnitus sufferer from Wynnewood, Pennsylvania. "And after 10 or 15 minutes, I'm totally refreshed. If I had any tinnitus when I began, it disappears."

Because tension in the jaw and neck area may aggravate tinnitus, learning how to control muscle spasms through biofeedback may also help. Some researchers are also studying the benefits of hypnosis as a tinnitus-management technique. In extreme cases, when nothing else helps, doctors may prescribe antianxiety or antidepression drugs (avoiding, of course, drugs that may be ototoxic).

Social Support ▶ Morris, president of the Delaware Valley Tinnitus Association, is actively involved in organizing tinnitus self-help groups in the Philadelphia area. The support of such groups, where tinnitus suf-

LOOKING FOR A CURE

Right now, there's no quick fix for tinnitus. But it may not be too long until doctors can prescribe a drug to silence the sounds altogether.

One of the most promising, yet preliminary, studies suggests that terfenadine—the common allergy drug commercially called Seldane—may partially or completely relieve tinnitus, even in people with no known allergies. Ronald G. Amedee, M.D., assistant professor of otolaryngology–head and neck surgery at Tulane Medical Center, gave 24 tinnitus patients a 60-milligram tablet twice a day for three 30-day periods. They were randomly assigned to receive Seldane during two of the 30-day blocks and a copycat placebo for the remaining period. Seventeen of the 24 showed some improvements in their tinnitus. And one of the 17—the only one with allergies who found relief with Seldane—saw it disappear altogether.

Dr. Amedee says it's not unusual to see tinnitus patients who have allergies respond to Seldane treatment. But this study may give hope to the non-allergic tinnitus sufferer. "Even subtle drops in the frequency or loudness of tinnitus are very important to those patients," he says. "Seldane may help them improve their quality of life."

Animal studies of tinnitus suggest that a certain calcium channel blocker used to decrease damage after a stroke may also be an effective treatment for tinnitus.

ferers can share their frustrations, successes and knowledge about the condition, may also help you get a handle on stress.

For more information, send $1 and a business-size, self-addressed envelope stamped with 75 cents to American Tinnitus Association, P.O. Box 5, Portland, OR 97207. Or call (503) 248-9985.

24   Routing Gout

*The "terrible toes" often can
be controlled with diet alone.*

Gout runs in Tom Lafavore's family. And when he's suffering a gout attack, it also runs—right down to his big toe, where tradition says it has paid back kings, nobles and rich men for thousands of years for their excesses.

Like most of the million other gout sufferers in America, Tom is not a nobleman, nor is he rich. He's a vocational-education teacher in Portland, Maine. But when gout first struck, he experienced a pain so excruciating that only a fellow gout sufferer would understand it, he says. "It's like constantly getting pounded on the toe with a sledgehammer." Twenty-four hours a day, for days on end.

Fortunately for all of you who suffer from this unique form of arthritis, the pain can be controlled—and you don't need a king's ransom to do it.

The Cause of Gout Is Crystal Clear

All gout attacks can be traced to a single problem: tiny crystals of uric acid that lodge in the lining of the joints and irritate them. Uric acid is one of our body's metabolic by-products. It's a kind of metabolic exhaust fume that the kidneys normally filter out and excrete through urine.

Many Americans have elevated levels of uric acid in their blood, either because there's too much for the kidneys to handle or because the kidneys aren't functioning properly. But only a small percentage of these people will ever have a gout attack. That's because the blood must become saturated with uric acid before crystal deposits begin to form in the joints.

"Think of what happens when you put too much

sugar in a glass of iced tea," says Jeffrey R. Lisse, M.D., director of the division of rheumatology at the University of Texas Medical Branch in Galveston. "The sugar will dissolve up to a point. Beyond that point the liquid can hold no more, and the remaining crystals pile up at the bottom. In gout, the excess crystals may pile up in the joints. What's not clear is why attacks are only intermittent although the crystals may be there for years."

Your First Bout with Gout

So you've just felt the first not-so-gentle twinges of stabbing joint pain. Is it gout? Or another form of arthritis? Check out these three distinctive warning signs of a gout attack. If you experience any of the signs and symptoms, be sure to pass the information on to your doctor.

Sign #1: Sudden Onset ▶ Gout strikes without warning—generally overnight—and quickly becomes very painful. Most other forms of arthritis begin gradually and get worse over several weeks or months, not several hours like gout.

Sign #2: Location, or "The Big-Toe Mystery" ▶ The first attack of gout strikes a single joint. More than half the time it wallops the big toe. In some cases, an ankle or knee is the initial battleground.

Scientists speculate that the lower joints are usually the ones to get hit because of gravity. Like sugar crystals in that glass of iced tea, the uric acid crystals settle to the bottom—and there's no place lower to go than your big toe. Previously injured joints are also more likely to be affected by gout. And there again, the big toe, ankle and knee, with all the banging about they get, remain likely candidates for a gout attack. (Exception: In older women who take diuretics, the first twinges may be felt in an elbow, wrist or finger.)

The affected joint usually looks swollen, and the skin turns deep red, as if infected. Later gout attacks may involve two or more joints, but the first attack rarely does.

Sign #3: Intensity ▶ Although the first attack may be relatively mild, sufferers swear there's no pain on earth like gout. "Older women with gout have told me that natural childbirth is less painful," says Robert Wortmann, M.D., professor of medicine and interim chairman of the Department of Medicine at the Medical College of Wisconsin.

Other forms of arthritis can be extraordinarily painful, too. But a little rest usually reduces the pain. Not so with gout. "It hurts constantly during an attack, no matter what I do," reports Tom. In fact, most people can't even tolerate the weight of a bed sheet on the affected area.

Getting the Gout Test

Gout or not, any sudden joint pain is cause for concern. Call your family physician or go to a hospital emergency room.

The doctor will ask about your risks and may order a blood test to check for high levels of uric acid. If your big toe is the affected spot, that may strongly suggest the diagnosis. But the only way to say for certain if it's gout is to check the inflamed joint for uric acid crystals.

The test is mercifully quick. After numbing the area with a supercold spray, the doctor removes fluid from the joint with a needle. The fluid is examined under a microscope for telltale crystals. Once the diagnosis is certain, treatment can begin.

Why do doctors insist on a proper diagnosis? Because it can save you a lot of pain—and perhaps the use of a limb. Certain drugs given for gout won't relieve other forms of arthritis. Delaying the proper treatment could cause permanent damage.

Five Steps That Lower Your Risk of Gout

No single risk factor is likely to put your big toe on red alert. But a combination of risk-raisers can trigger an

211
■

all-out gout attack. Fortunately, you can lower some of those risks by taking the following steps.

Lose Weight, Yes... ▶ Doctors say that more than half of all gout patients are overweight. And the greater your girth, the more susceptible you are to chronic diseases that can alter uric acid concentrations in the blood. Tom's experience bears this out: He's a diet-controlled diabetic, a factor doctors say increases his risk.

...But Don't Crash Diet! ▶ If you have some weight to lose, don't go on a crash diet. The shock to your metabolism can raise uric acid levels and trigger gout. "Twice, I've had gout attacks while I was trying to lose a lot of weight," says Tom. "Even my antigout medication didn't prevent one of the episodes." The moral: Lose weight gradually with a sensible low-fat diet and exercise.

Don't Overindulge ▶ Purine is a protein by-product that is used by the body during cell growth or repair. When purines are burned up, the end product is uric acid. People prone to gout are often told to go on a low-purine diet to reduce uric acid buildup.

"That's been overrated. The best diet for most gout sufferers is a weight-loss diet," says Herbert S. Diamond, M.D., clinical professor of medicine at the University of Pittsburgh and chairman of the Department of Medicine at Western Pennsylvania Hospital. Purine-rich foods—like organ meats, gravies, anchovies, herring and sardines—may trigger an attack in people with high uric acid levels, but others can tolerate them in small portions.

Cut the Alcohol ▶ In gout, what you drink is more important than what you eat. Alcohol is doubly bad: It increases uric acid production and interferes with the kidneys' ability to filter it out—no matter how much urine you may pass. People at risk don't have to give up the occasional toast, but overdoing it tempts fate.

Drink Water Instead ▶ Water can help flush uric acid out of your system. That old H_2O also helps maintain the fluid volume in your bloodstream. (Gout attacks can be triggered by dehydration in high-risk people.) You can easily maintain your fluid intake by drinking a 12-ounce glass of water or juice with every meal.

Actually, any shock that reduces the volume of blood or revs up the body's repair systems can raise uric acid levels and cause gout: sudden serious illness, surgery, even too much exercise. Fixing the primary problem will clear up the gout.

Some beneficial medicines can trigger gout, too. The most common culprits are diuretics, often prescribed for high blood pressure, heart failure or fluid retention. It's important to consult your doctor at the first sign of diuretic-induced gout. Don't stop taking the medication on your own!

Put That Gout to Rout

If left untreated, your first attack of gout can last five to ten days. After that, it goes away on its own.

However, there's no reason to wait. Quick intervention with anti-inflammatory drugs can parry an attack within 24 hours.

The treatment of choice for an acute gout attack is any one of the many nonsteroidal anti-inflammatory drugs (NSAIDs). Most NSAIDs are extremely effective and cause only mild side effects: stomach upset, headache, skin rashes and, on rare occasions, ulcers. The most popular antigout NSAIDs are indomethacin and naproxen. Both are available only by prescription. Nonprescription ibuprofen is also used.

The great-great-grandpa of antigout medicines is an anti-inflammatory called colchicine (*COAL-chih-seen*). Plant extracts containing colchicine were used to fight gout over 1,500 years ago. In all that time, no one has figured out exactly how it works. But work it does, especially when taken during the first two days of an attack.

Colchicine has lost ground to the NSAIDs because it takes a toll on people's digestive tracts: About 80 percent of patients will experience diarrhea, nausea and stomach cramps as side effects. Injecting colchicine into a vein can bypass stomach problems, but it requires a trip to the doctor. Despite these drawbacks, colchicine is still prescribed for those who don't respond well to the NSAIDs. It comes in a prescription-only tablet, usually taken in several small daily doses.

In some cases, doctors will inject a corticosteroid directly into the affected joint to reduce pain and swelling. But one major side effect severely limits the usefulness of this treatment: If a single joint undergoes more than three injections, there's a risk of tendon and ligament damage. So corticosteroids are a last resort.

Fighting Future Attacks

First-time gout patients should be optimistic. A majority of these people will never suffer another attack. You can increase your odds of being in that majority by following some of the preventive measures mentioned earlier: Lose weight slowly, and drink more water and much less alcohol.

Some patients at high risk of a second gout attack won't actually have one until years later. Formerly, these people would have been put on antigout drugs for life. But now doctors tend to take a wait-and-see attitude. Patients are given a bottle of colchicine or prescription nonsteroidal anti-inflammatory drugs, with instructions to take some at the first sign of an attack.

Attacking Gout at Its Roots

Ultimately, only 25 percent of people who get gout will need a permanent prescription to prevent or reduce future attacks. Patients aren't generally put in this category until they've had three or more gout attacks within a year. The drugs used for long-term management fight the cause of gout, not the symptoms: These drugs are useless against pain and swelling during an attack. The preferred drug for the veteran of gout is allopurinol. It actually slows the rate at which your body produces uric acid.

Allopurinol is the best medicine for people with uric

acid stones or other kidney problems because it reduces the kidneys' work load. It may reduce your work load, too, since it makes a minority of patients drowsy or less alert.

Patients who can't tolerate allopurinol are given an older class of medicine, the uricosuric drugs. The best-known of these drugs is probenecid. Kidneys get no breaks here: Uricosurics work by increasing the amount of uric acid passed in the urine. Early on, people taking these drugs must drink liberal amounts of fluid to keep their urine diluted, or they'll get kidney stones.

Uricosurics are preferred in some cases for their ability to help dissolve painful deposits of uric acid crystals that accumulate over time. In uncontrolled gout, these deposits can cause irreversible damage to the joints and form disfiguring lumps under the skin and in the cartilage of the ear.

Both allopurinol and uricosurics are taken orally, and they have similar side effects. Both can cause stomach upset, which generally goes away after the body becomes accustomed to the drug. They also can cause skin rashes, which in rare cases can become a serious problem.

Ironically, both drugs can increase the frequency of gout attacks during the first six months of use. Doctors think that reducing blood uric acid levels so quickly causes the crystals to move around inside the joints. To control this cruel twist of fate, most patients take low doses of colchicine or NSAIDs for several months after starting treatment.

Once begun, allopurinol or a uricosuric must usually be taken for life. (New research suggests that some people— particularly those of normal weight—may be able to decrease their need for medication over time.) Talk over your medication options with your doctor. Tom Lafavore did. "I'm currently taking allopurinol, and for me it's worth it.

"In six years I've had only two additional gout attacks. And at least one of those attacks was caused by skipping my medicine. So stick with it," he advises.

For more information about gout or any other form of arthritis, contact your local Arthritis Foundation chapter or write to the national office at P.O. Box 19000, Atlanta, GA 30326. Or call the Arthritis Foundation Information Line toll-free at (800) 283-7800.

215

Emotional Fitness

When Love Goes Cold

25

Rekindle desire when the fire's gone out of your relationship.

By Jennifer Knopf, Ph.D.,
and Michael Seiler, Ph.D.

Perhaps you have heard the joke, "How many therapists does it take to change a light bulb?"

The answer: "One, but the light bulb really has to want to change."

Part of what makes people laugh at a joke like this is the element of truth that they can find in it. When it comes to the problem doctors call inhibited sexual desire (ISD)—a lack of interest in sex, or an inability to feel sexual or get sexually aroused—the truth is that you and your partner must really want to rebuild your sexual relationship in order to attempt the effort that will be asked of you.

Some of our patients—like Wendy, whose interest in sex had not bounced back two years after her husband's death, and Larry, who had felt no sexual desire since suffering a heart attack—are painfully aware of their own ISD and its impact on their lives. They know that they want to restore their sexual desire. You may fit this description as well.

Other patients—like Andrea and Paul, who were dissatisfied with the frequency and quality of their lovemaking, and Bobby, who was baffled by his lack of interest in sex—have struggled to integrate sexuality into their lives and relationships. They want to change so that sex can be a pleasure rather than the void it now is. That may be what you want, too.

Detecting Barriers to Change

217

No matter what ISD has taken from you—closeness, sexual pleasure, a source of relaxation or stimulation, self-confidence or positive feelings about your partner—you may have also gained something from it. You may wonder what you could gain by losing interest in sex.

What good could possibly come from something that has probably driven a wedge between you and your partner; that has saddled one or both of you with hurt, angry or resentful feelings; that has left you anxious, insecure or feeling inadequate, and wreaked havoc on your self-esteem and your relationship?

The answer is that ISD may help you avoid situations that you find more threatening than your present circumstances.

If you want to find out what ISD may be protecting you from, simply ask yourself: "What negative outcomes might result from increasing my or my partner's interest in sex?"

Could your relationship be getting too close for comfort, suffocating you, or paving the way for your partner to make more demands than you could meet? If your partner becomes more interested in sex, will you need to face your own performance anxieties and sense of inadequacy? If you start to feel sexual desire, what will you have to give up in order to find time in your overcrowded schedule to have sex? And if you are often pushed around by a domineering partner, what will you have left to help you even the score or reassure yourself that you have some power in your relationship? Not having ISD could mean the loss of a powerful bargaining tool that helps influence or control your partner's behavior. These are the kinds of consequences that many of our patients fear more than those of having ISD or relating to a partner who has it.

A serious but hidden relationship problem may also present a barrier to change. Camouflaged by a litany of minor conflicts and small complaints, more fundamental and frightening issues may stand between you and a more satisfying sex life. These include lack of trust, fear of intimacy or rejection, old anger and resentment, or unfinished business from your past. You maintain the smokescreen of arguments and minor skirmishes, both because the underlying problem is affecting your feelings about yourself or your partner and because one or both of you fear that acknowledging the underlying problem will ultimately destroy your self-esteem or your relationshi.

Couples in therapy are often able to confront and de. with those problems immediately. On the other hand, you may feel the effect of underlying issues without quite knowing what they are. Because this happens so often, we will discuss some common signs of resistance to change or sexual sabotage and ways to handle them. However, if you find that you cannot get moving again, we recommend that you seek professional help in the form of marital counseling or sex therapy, or both.

Another barrier is assuming that your sexual problem is a medical one and that, as a result, there is nothing you can do about it. While some sexual disorders, including ISD, are caused by physical factors or medical conditions, this is not a conclusion you should draw prematurely or without professional advice. If you suspect that there is a connection between ISD and a physical problem, a medical evaluation—including a thorough physical examination and laboratory tests—can confirm or rule out your theory. If your assumption proves incorrect, as it did for Larry, who believed his heart attack had altered his body chemistry and destroyed his sex drive, you will need to confront the emotional and interpersonal barriers that are currently blocking your sexual desire.

If there is a medical reason for your sexual problem, there may be a medical treatment for it as well. And even if there isn't, you can still learn to engage in satisfying sexual activities and improve your sexual relationship. A physical condition, no matter what it is, may limit the range of what you can do sexually, but it does not mean you cannot be sexual at all.

Another barrier that we often encounter with our ISD patients is too much anger. There is a good chance that this barrier is operating in your relationship if:

■ Your attempts at communication quickly lead to knock-down, drag-out fights with a lot of yelling, screaming, criticizing or even throwing things.

219
∎

■ The angry feelings you or your partner express are out of control or an overreaction to the situation at hand.

■ Bitter, hurtful arguments are repeated time and time again but never seem to resolve the problems that lead to them.

■ Resentful, hurt and angry feelings linger long after the argument ends.

■ One partner's passive anger blocks communication. More difficult to identify than the explosive fury we just described, quiet anger takes the form of withdrawal, "forgetting," coldness, being subtly uncooperative or blatantly doing the exact opposite of what is asked, walking away from a conversation or otherwise creating a silence that cannot be broken.

Regardless of the form it takes, if you and your partner cannot get beyond your anger, you will not be able to solve your sexual problem—and on some level you will not want to. You may have to work through the relationship problems—perhaps with the help of a psychotherapist—before you can tackle the sexual ones.

Finally, a barrier we often observe in one partner is the tendency to avoid admitting you really do have a problem. You may believe that acknowledging sexual problems of any kind, and sexual desire disorders in particular, is an admission of personal failure and inadequacy.

ISD and the conflicts it causes will not go away just because you don't pay attention to them, however. In fact, your own or your partner's distress and dissatisfaction will probably escalate, until you can no longer ignore them because you are in too much pain. We can only hope that while reading this you have decided to stop burying your head in the sand and are willing to take steps to solve your problem now, rather than waiting for a severe crisis to force you to change.

Prerequisites for Rekindling Desire

Before you actually attempt the self-help steps we have provided, there are several things you must do to create a climate that is conducive to change. The ability to express your needs, thoughts and feelings without blaming or attacking your partner, to listen and confirm that you understand what your partner is saying, to respond without becoming defensive and to negotiate differences of opinion effectively is essential for solving day-to-day problems. These skills will also help you broach the subject of ISD with your partner. Consequently, we would like to offer you the following tips.

Recognize that both you and your partner have the right to express your needs, thoughts, feelings and concerns. This right brings with it the responsibility to present your point of view in the manner that is least likely to hurt or provoke the other person.

Say what you mean. Express yourself clearly and directly. Do not beat around the bush, saying one thing when you mean something else or watering down your feelings (saying you are "a little concerned" about your sex life, for instance, when you are actually extremely upset about it and frightened that your relationship is coming to an end). Clearly identify your feelings, explain what you are thinking, specify what is bothering you, and let your partner know what you need as directly as possible. This is vital when discussing ISD. Saying "Our sex life stinks, and you can either shape up or ship out, buddy" is definitely direct, but it is neither specific nor helpful. "I'm unhappy having sex only once a month, and I'd like to talk about what we could do to have it more often than that" is both more to the point and more likely to pave the way for a productive discussion.

Use "I" messages to express your feelings, beliefs, needs and wishes. For example, say "I get upset when I find dirty dishes in the sink," or "I need you to help me by cleaning up the kitchen after you get a snack," instead of "You are a hopeless slob," or "You like making messes for me to clean up, don't you?" "I" statements express what you are feeling while breaking the pattern of making accusations or generalizations.

Make a concerted effort not to begin conversations or statements with "You always" or "You never." Such generalizations are rarely true, and they only invite a coun-

221

terattack. For instance, when discussing ISD, you are much more likely to make progress by saying "I feel pressured and frustrated when you come on to me at the end of a rough day, and I wish you could be more sensitive to how stressed out I am sometimes" than if you say "You're a selfish, insensitive bum who never stops to think about how I'm feeling before you demand that I drop everything and have sex with you."

Listen attentively. Focus your attention on what is being said to you, not on what you are going to say in response.

Listen actively. After your partner finishes speaking, reflect the message you heard, summarizing or paraphrasing what you think your partner said. Clarify by asking if that is what your partner meant and if you might have missed anything. Respond by expressing your feelings about your partner's message as well as your ideas about the topic being discussed.

Remember that neither of you is a mind reader. Do not assume that your partner understands your point of view or that you understand your partner's thoughts or feelings. You should also definitely avoid voicing your partner's thoughts or feelings—as in "You think that my job isn't as important as yours," or "You're not really angry about the dirty dishes. You're still trying to make me feel guilty about stopping to have a drink with the guys."

Focus discussions. When communicating in general or for the purpose of solving a problem, making a decision or negotiating a compromise:

■ Discuss one topic at a time, focusing your attention on that area and how it affects each of you here and now. Do not kitchen-sink (bring up other current problems or old business from previous conflicts).

■ Skip the question of whose fault it is that the problem exists. Blaming your partner and justifying or defending your own behavior will not help. In fact, you should try to acknowledge your own part in the situation and identify what you are willing to do to resolve it.

■ Make sure you have enough uninterrupted time to discuss the matter.

■ Be specific about what the problem or subject under discussion is.

■ Move toward a win/win outcome, one in which both of you get at least some of what you need, rather than having one partner's needs met at the other's expense.

Practice on the easy topics first. If communication between you and your partner has been strained and ineffective in the past, practice this new approach with topics that are relatively easy to discuss before tackling the emotionally charged issues.

When Your Partner Resists Change

Even if you follow the guidelines above, there is no guarantee that your partner will agree to work on the problem or even admit that there is a problem. In fact, your partner may steadfastly refuse all suggestions for change. If this occurs, you may feel hurt or angry, or you may jump to the conclusion that your partner simply does not love you and wants your relationship to end. But this is only sometimes the case. So before you let your imagination run away with you, try to put yourself in your partner's shoes, considering that one of the barriers to change may be making it hard to face the situation.

More often than not, we find that resistant partners, especially if they are the ones with ISD, are acutely aware of the problem and feel terrible about it. Unfortunately, either they are convinced it cannot be fixed or they are frightened that trying to change will reveal aspects of themselves or their relationship that they will be unable to handle.

We suggest that you give your partner time to think about the situation and your requests, especially if your concerns come as a surprise. Perhaps you could give your

223
■

partner this chapter to read. Then, in a few days or weeks, try again to start another discussion and see if some change can occur.

If your partner continues to resist, you will eventually have to confront the consequences of not working together to improve the situation. You might say something like "If we can't work together to solve this problem, then I can't feel good about you or our relationship. It makes me wonder what our relationship means to you, and maybe I have to rethink my commitment to the relationship, too. I'm not sure what sort of answers I'll come up with, but if we can't agree to do something together, I'm going to have to find a solution I can live with."

You may have to present more specific consequences as well, letting your partner know that if you cannot work things out between you, then you want to get into therapy together, or separate temporarily, or get divorced. Do not make threats you do not intend to carry out, however, or hurl ultimatums that do more harm than good. Many higher-desire partners have vowed to have an affair and have even gone through with it, only to discover that they are even farther from a resolution to their marital and sexual problems.

Realize as well that if your partner will not change, and you cannot learn to live with the situation as it is, separation or divorce may, in fact, become a realistic alternative. However, this rarely occurs because of a sexual-desire problem alone.

In addition, although it won't necessarily change your relationship or your sex life, until your partner is ready to work with you, you can work on changing yourself, improving your self-esteem and increasing your options for the future.

Deciding What You Really Want

As you come to terms with your sexual problems and your need for change, you and your partner must individually and jointly set goals for yourselves. You need to clarify what you want from each other, your overall relationship and, specifically, your sex life—and your goals in all three areas must be reasonable. They must take into consideration the realities of your lifestyle as well as your partner's needs and wishes.

The following self-help steps can help in this area. They can also allow you to establish a mutually agreeable contract for change.

You will need at least one hour's worth of time per partner, possibly spread over several days, to clarify and set your own goals individually, and as much time as it takes to agree on mutual goals.

What do you want more or less of in your sex life? In your relationship? From your partner? Working alone, you and your partner should make separate lists answering these questions for yourselves in a general way. For example, answers might include frequent sexual interactions, more sex play before intercourse, more variety during sex, less pressure to have sex, more communication, more help around the house, bringing less work home from the office, more time for just the two of you and so on. You need not complete the list in one sitting.

Next, choose the two or three items from each category that are most important to you. Then, for each item or goal you have chosen, write specific examples of what you would ideally want in that area and the bare minimum you would accept in that area.

State these goals in the most precise terms possible, with your ideal reflecting how things would turn out under the best of all possible circumstances. This is your "wish list" and does not have to reflect the realities of your current lifestyle.

Your minimum expectation should be somewhere between where things are now and your goal. Your minimum should represent the least amount of change you would settle for.

For example, Barbara wanted to have sex more often. Her ideal was "To be able to have intercourse whenever I am in the mood for it." Her minimum was "To have intercourse at least three times a month." Her husband, Dan, on the other hand, wanted less pressure to have sex. His ideal was "No sexual pressure from Barbara. She would let me decide when to have sex." His minimum was "She could ask for sex whenever she felt like it but would be more accepting of me when I wasn't in the mood."

Set a reasonable standard to work toward—by identifying a goal that falls somewhere between your ideal and your bare minimum. Barbara's goal, for instance, was to have intercourse once a week, while Dan's was to be approached for sex no more than twice a week, to not be approached when Barbara knew he was under work pressure and to retain the right to refuse Barbara's sexual overtures.

After setting such goals, you and your partner must negotiate and compromise to establish goals you can agree to work together to achieve. Once you have set your own realistic standards, sit down together and compare lists. Try to find a middle ground on similar goals. For instance, Barbara and Dan compromised in this way by agreeing to work toward having sex three to four times a month. Barbara agreed to make sexual overtures only when she felt a very strong desire to have sex, while also considering how much stress Dan might be under at the time. Although Dan retained the right to refuse any sexual invitation, he agreed to tell Barbara why he was refusing and to work on stress and time management so that he could be more receptive to her advances.

Negotiate trade-offs—giving your partner something he or she wants in exchange for something you want—even though one goal may have nothing to do with the other.

Considering the complexity of such agreements, four points are worth making. First, negotiating your contract for change will take some time and effort and will require you to follow the discussion guidelines we mentioned. Second, although your agreement is not carved in granite and can be renegotiated at any time, you will find it helpful to write down what you have agreed to do. Third, if you find your partner does not follow through on part of the bargain, we recommend that you follow through on your part anyway. Fourth, both of you must recognize and accept that you will not reach your goals immediately. Look for progress, not overnight turnarounds.

As long as both of you are working toward those goals, you are sticking to your contract. However, if either or both of you behave in ways that clearly keep you from moving toward your goals, you must discuss the situation right away and, if necessary, get outside help.

This strategy reflects the obvious but so often overlooked reality that both partners in an intimate relationship will get more of what they want if each is willing to give the other more of what he or she wants.

Smoothing the Way to Success

This whole process of communicating, goal setting and regaining intimacy will be a lot smoother if you:

1. Use the strong, positive areas of your relationship as building blocks. When rearranging your schedule, try not to let go of the activities that help you and your partner enjoy each other or feel close emotionally. In fact, try to increase these behaviors, focusing as much as possible on your own and your partner's good points.

2. Try to increase physical contact in general. Do more touching, hugging and hand-holding. Scratch his back, massage her hands or head. Simply enjoy being physically close for its own sake, not as a prelude to sex.

3. Add a bit of romance to your lifestyle. Have special dinners, remember special days, dress up and go out to dinner even if you're only going to the local pizza parlor. Leave notes, send cards, give gifts, bring home flowers just for the joy of it. Get away once in a while, whether to a romantic Caribbean island or to a motel three miles from your home. Create a romantic environment for the self-help exercise and when having sex. Try candlelight, music, silk sheets, exotic fragrances and so on.

4. Be playful and creative. Do something surprising, like wearing a sexy new outfit. Come up with imaginative ways to spend time together. Do things together that you

227

did when you first dated. Stir up some nostalgia by looking through old photos or visiting the places you fre-
quented while you were dating. Forget about mowing the
lawn or cleaning out the hall closet and take a drive in
the country. Try some activity together that you've never
tried before. You'll find that putting the adult in you on
hold for a bit can be beneficial for both your relationship
and your sex life.

26   Breathe Free

How to de-stress your life—
one breath at a time.

For 20 minutes, you sit quietly as your co-workers
make their presentations before a packed house. Now it's
your turn. You rise and slowly make your way to the
podium. With each step your anxiety level climbs. By the
time you reach the microphone, your palms are moist,
your muscles are tight, and your breathing is short and
shallow. You can actually feel your pulse pounding in
your ear.

You're experiencing your body's automatic stress
response—that built-in survival mechanism designed to
pump you up for action when danger threatens. But
when—instead of battling it out or running away—you've
got to stand and deliver, it sure would be nice if you could
switch off the pump.

Unfortunately, you can't consciously slow your heartbeat or shut off your body's sweat glands. But you can
throw the stress response in reverse. Simply start by
breathing slowly and deeply. "Breathing is one of the
body's mechanisms that you can control when you want
to," says Guylaine Coté, Ph.D., at the Center for Stress and
Anxiety Disorders at the State University of New York
(SUNY) at Albany. "Taking slow, deep breaths reduces
the flood of fight-or-flight symptoms, dropping blood
pressure, slowing pulse rate and relaxing tense muscles."

The respiratory response in a stressful situation—to gulp short and fast—is called "overbreathing" by the experts. It induces additional feelings of anxiety. It prevents sufficient oxygen from making it to the brain, causing you to feel dizzy, light-headed and confused—maybe even blurring your vision. The heart speeds up to pump more blood, and as sweat breaks out on your upper lip, another physiological effect—the constriction of blood vessels—is turning your hands to ice.

The quickest way to stop the physiological landslide—and conserve your energy for better things—is to correct the poor breathing as soon as it's detected.

Precisely because of its calming effect, using one's own breath is a cornerstone treatment in stress reduction and pain-control programs around the country.

It's also a fundamental part of yoga—an ancient practice that a lot of very modern, stressed-out people swear by. The combination of conscious breathing, focused relaxation and stretching exercises makes yoga one of the most tranquilizing do-it-yourself de-stressors around.

Yoga Breathing

Deep abdominal, or diaphragmatic, breathing simply means that the diaphragm should be engaged—it's the large dome-shaped muscle that arches upward and across the base of the lungs. When a person inhales deeply, the diaphragm contracts, allowing more air into the lung's lower lobes.

Breathing diaphragmatically has the added bonus of relaxing the muscles of the torso. "Tightness in the stomach, chest and rib cage spontaneously relaxes when you breathe deeply," explains Patricia Hammond, instructor with the American Yoga Association, in Sarasota, Florida.

To distinguish between diaphragmatic and chest breathing for yourself, place your hand on your belly, a little above the navel. This is the area—not your chest—that should expand when you inhale. Try to breathe in so that your hand rises. It will probably feel unnatural at first. That's okay. It takes one to two weeks of regular practice (twice a day for ten-minute stints) to get the hang of abdominal breathing.

A more advanced deep-breathing technique is known as the "three-part breath," also called the "yogic complete breath." Begin as before, by first expanding the abdomen. As you continue to inhale, allow the air to expand upward into the midchest area. Then, fill the upper chest so that your collarbones start to lift. Continue inhaling until your lungs are filled to capacity. When you exhale, reverse the order, deflating from top to bottom.

Once deep, abdominal breathing feels comfortable and natural, the next step is learning to breathe more slowly. At the SUNY clinic this is accomplished by focusing the attention on the breath by counting.

Begin by saying "one" to yourself, followed by a slow inhalation (at least three seconds). Breathing through your nose will give you better control of the breath, making it slower and smoother. After full expansion, pause and think "relax." Then exhale. Exhalations should be three seconds or longer. At the end of the exhalation, pause and say "two." Inhale again, and so on. At some point, time yourself to see if you match the recommended rate of 10 to 14 breaths per minute rather than the more common 16 to 18.

Dr. Coté recommends "minipractices" of diaphragmatic breathing whenever you become aware that your breathing is irregular.

Yoga Relaxation

Yoga's conscious relaxation of muscles and internal awareness are common components of several stress-reduction techniques. Patients at the University of Massachusetts Medical Center's stress-reduction clinic learn to identify their own hot spots with a yogic technique called the "body scan." To perform the body scan, lie on your back, close your eyes, and simply breathe. After a few minutes, start at the bottom left and concentrate on each body part: toes, foot, calf, knee, front thigh, back thigh, hip. Repeat to the right, and then move up the torso, arms and head.

As you focus completely on each point, note the sensations and imagine your breath going in and out of each area. Imagine releasing the weight of each part, feeling it "melt" right into the floor.

"The subtle benefit of practicing this type of exercise is that people become more aware of their body on a daily basis," says Hammond. "Then even when they're sitting at their desk at work, they'll notice, 'Oh, my stomach's tense' or 'I'm clenching my teeth.' The simple act of bringing awareness to the tense area will allow you to release it using the techniques you've learned."

Yoga Stretches

"The stronger and healthier your body is, the less pain and stress you'll suffer in general," says Jon Kabat-Zinn, Ph.D., director of the stress program at the University of Massachusetts Medical Center and author of *Full-Catastrophe Living.*

Yoga stretches are poses or postures with names like lotus, tree and frog. Although a stretch should never be painful, it's not always easy, either. But the long-term outcome is positive. Over a period of months you develop greater flexibility. In turn, the muscles respond by lengthening.

Yoga postures are best learned from an experienced teacher, since precision and proper alignment make the difference between so-so and superb benefits—in addition to reducing the risk of muscle and joint injury.

For a taste of yoga, however, the following warm-up sequence should be gentle enough for just about anyone to try at home. (Check first with your doctor if you have any low back, neck or serious medical problem.) In general, take complete inhalations before you move, then exhale slowly as you move into postures. Breathe normally while holding a posture or in between. Never hold your breath unless directed to do so.

■ Begin with a resting pose. Lie on your back, arms at your sides, palms up. Close your eyes and imagine the floor supporting the weight of your body—arms, legs,

231

torso, head. Take several "three-part breaths," then let your breathing flow naturally.

■ From here, move into the "knee squeeze." First, inhale slowly and fully. As you begin to exhale, bring your right knee to your chest, wrapping your hands around it. Gently lift your head to your knee, squeezing the knee toward you. Upon inhalation, lower the leg back to the floor. Repeat on the left side. Pause, taking some normal breaths.

■ Inhale, and as you exhale bring both knees to the chest. Inhale while holding, and move on the exhale, lifting your head toward your knees. (If you don't have back problems, you may wish to do a few "spinal rocks," rocking gently forward and back, breathing naturally.) Inhale as you lower your head and legs back to the floor.

■ While lying on your back, stretch your arms over your head, your hands touching the floor. As you begin to

HOW TO FIND
A GOOD YOGA CLASS

If you feel ready for a limber body and more peace of mind and would like to give yoga a try, keep the following tips in mind when looking for a class.

Ask others for their opinions. Says Steven Brena, M.D., chairman of the board at the Pain Control and Rehabilitation Institute of Georgia, "Ask the people who have experienced a certain technique, 'What are the results of your practice?' 'Are you happy with the class?' "

Inquire about the style before signing up. There are numerous different "styles" of yoga, not all of which emphasize relaxation. While most styles do incorporate relaxation techniques, some are downright strenuous. Check with the instructor up front before making assumptions.

inhale, stretch your right foot out, pointing your toe, and reach your left arm away from your head, fingers spread apart. Stretch as far as you can. Release, exhaling, and imagine that all bodily tension is leaving through your breath. Repeat with the opposite arm and leg. After several rounds, lie still and enjoy the sensations.

■ Next, lying on your back, bend your knees, keeping them together, and rest your feet on the floor. Clasp your hands behind your head, elbows to the floor. Inhale deeply. As you exhale, slowly lower your legs to the floor on the right. Rest in this position, breathing naturally. Try to keep the left arm as close to the floor as possible, feeling the gentle stretch in the spine. Inhale and bring the legs back to center. Repeat on the left side.

■ Complete the cycle by returning to the resting pose, focusing on the nice sensations that stretching has aroused in your body.

Look for a teacher who individualizes instruction. Everybody's different, and instructors should adapt exercises to accommodate your arthritis, low back problem or other physical concern.

If you can, take a trial class before you invest long-term. An instructor who's concerned with meeting your needs will allow you to get a taste before you slap down payment for a year-long stint.

Be suspicious of an institute that asks for a lot of money. Yoga classes are offered by many YMCAs and independent teachers. Average prices range from $5 to $15 for a group session to up to $20 to $30 for private lessons. Some yoga institutes hold weekend and week-long retreats that may include meals and lectures on health and nutrition, which are, of course, more expensive.

233

For Best Results

When practicing yoga, you need to keep a few points in mind.

"At the very least, you need to know that you should not compete," says Martin Pierce, director of the Pierce Program, a yoga studio based in Atlanta, Georgia. "If you are looking around at others thinking you must do as well as they do, you are going to create more stress for yourself." The way to experience inner relaxation is to direct your attention inward.

In the same vein, yoga at best is non-goal-oriented. "If you are trying really hard to relax, you won't relax," says Prescott, Arizona, imagery consultant Annabelle Nelson, Ph.D.

And you must be willing to practice regularly. "People can't expect to benefit greatly from yoga without making a commitment to it," says Dr. Kabat-Zinn.

While the deepest benefits of yoga occur with commitment over time, newcomers are likely to experience a welcome tranquillity during the very first lesson.

Do
It
Naturally

Arthritis Options 27

Questions and answers about some unconventional therapies.

By Fred G. Kantrowitz, M.D.

Unconventional therapy is therapy that has not been scientifically proven to be effective. This does not always mean the treatment has not been tested, nor does it mean the results have not been positive. It simply means there haven't been enough tests to assure the treatment is sound. Fish oil is an example. Although a few studies have shown that this may be of value in the treatment of rheumatoid arthritis, a lot of work remains to be done before it can be classified as an accepted treatment option.

Of much more concern are treatments that have not been adequately studied. It has been estimated that between $1 billion and $2 billion a year is spent on unproven remedies, most of which involve unproven arthritis remedies ranging from the harmless, such as wearing a copper bracelet, to the potentially dangerous. Why do some people persist in their belief that a certain therapy works, even if there is no scientific evidence to validate their perception?

First, coincidences do happen, and since there are 37 million arthritis sufferers in the United States, there is a lot of opportunity for these to occur. Also, since arthritis is an extremely variable disease, it is easy to attach inappropriate significance to a new treatment. The arthritis may have been getting better anyway.

Second is the placebo response, which means you have a positive response to a treatment, such as the classic sugar pill, that should not work. This can be construed as an example of positive thinking—if you think something will work, it will. As many as one-third of individuals exposed to a placebo note improvement afterward.

The most common questions regarding unconventional therapy follow. Some answers may prove surprising—there may be something to some of these cures after all.

Q: Is there anything I can add to my diet to improve my arthritis?

A: Patients have added a myriad of substances to their diets in the hope of controlling their arthritis. One of the most popular has been cod-liver oil, the folk theory being that it helps lubricate joints. There is no evidence that this therapy is effective. But other types of fish oils are being studied, and preliminary findings indicate they may be of some benefit in the treatment of rheumatoid arthritis.

Fish oil contains the polyunsaturated acids eicosapentaenoic acid (EPA) and docosahexaenoic acid (DHA), which are termed omega-3 fatty acids. It is these acids that may produce improvement in patients with rheumatoid arthritis. Although cod-liver oil contains these acids, it is also rich in vitamins A and D (which can be dangerous if taken in large amounts) and cholesterol. Cod-liver oil is therefore an inappropriate source of fish oil.

Although fish oil's effect on rheumatoid arthritis is seldom dramatic, it appears sufficiently safe to warrant being tried in addition to your regular treatment—not instead of it—if your physician so recommends.

A reasonable approach is to increase consumption of fish rich in omega-3 fatty acids. These include oily, cold saltwater fish such as tuna, salmon, mackerel and sardines, among others.

Q: What about other kinds of doctors, such as chiropractors and osteopaths? Can they help?

A: Studies show that, in patients with musculoskeletal problems, chiropractic adjustments provide quicker pain relief than a placebo. After a few weeks, however, the benefits appear to cease. When manipulation is compared with massage techniques, it works more quickly. However, within six to seven weeks, the benefits appear equal.

Thus, if manipulation does help, it should be used early, and it makes little sense to use it for prolonged periods of time. Its effects may be transitory, and patients sometimes feel worse after a treatment session.

Despite the perceived (and real) antagonism between physicians and chiropractors, many practitioners of the two disciplines recognize what the other has to offer and even refer patients to one another. It's important for all concerned to keep an open mind, especially when a patient's arthritis isn't improving.

Doctors of osteopathic medicine (osteopaths, or D.O.'s) have training similar to traditional doctors—they prescribe medication and perform surgery—but they also believe in the importance of spinal manipulation and perform this procedure in addition to traditional techniques.

Q: What about acupuncture?

A: Again, we should be open-minded. Acupuncture occasionally appears capable of reducing the pain of arthritis but not the inflammation. Thus, continued joint damage may ensue. There is no concrete evidence that it is an adequate treatment for arthritis, especially over the long run. Even in China, other forms of therapy, including traditional Western approaches, are used to treat the arthritic patient.

Despite this, acupuncture is sometimes helpful, and if you decide to try it, go to a bona fide acupuncturist, not a Western M.D. who isn't completely trained in the discipline.

Ironically, traditional Western medicine has incorporated techniques similar to those of chiropractic medicine and acupuncture. Physical therapists occasionally perform manipulation and also utilize acupressure and electrical stimulation, both of which are similar in theory to acupuncture.

Just remember, acupuncture and chiropractic techniques are not substitutes for a complete medical evaluation and should be utilized only with the advice and consent of your physician. I've seen too many patients who thought they had "routine" low back pain and went for acupuncture or spinal manipulation and were eventually discovered to have much more serious problems—including cancer.

239

Q: Is there any benefit to yoga?

A: Some yoga exercises are similar to range-of-motion exercises taught by physical therapists. Yoga exercises are performed slowly while practicing deep-breathing techniques. Force and stress are not involved, and there are no bouncing, jerky motions. In a sense, yoga exercises are the opposite of high-impact aerobic exercises, which are good for keeping in shape but do not offer any benefit to your joints. Although yoga appears to be rather safe on the whole, some of the advanced positions can put extra stress on the joints and should be avoided.

Patients with arthritis often find the exercises beneficial and claim that yoga also provides a means of relaxing and reducing stress.

Although not yet scrutinized by Western statistical analysis, yoga appears sufficiently safe and potentially helpful to warrant giving it a try if you are so inclined. It is not a substitute for traditional medical and physical-therapy approaches but can be used to supplement them. Indeed, some patients carry over the principles of yoga to their physical-therapy programs and claim to be much the better for using the combination.

Q: I heard that DMSO is a good treatment for arthritis. What is it, and is this true?

A: There is no evidence that DMSO, or dimethyl sulfoxide, is anything but a mild pain-reliever. It is usually available in a veterinary strength not intended for human use. Skin rashes, headache, nausea and diarrhea can result from its use. It also produces a garliclike taste in the mouth. It is applied topically and given intravenously.

Clinics have sprung up that administer this drug. Patients are encouraged to return frequently, as often as three or four times a week, and often at great expense. There is nothing to suggest this approach is helpful. In fact, it is potentially harmful because side effects may result and more reliable treatments may be ignored.

Q: Radiation is used to treat other serious diseases. Can it be used to treat arthritis?

A: X-ray therapy directed to the spine was once used to treat ankylosing spondylitis but has now been abandoned, in part because of the subsequent development of malignancies.

More recently, radiation directed to the lymph nodes has been used to treat rheumatoid arthritis. The rationale behind this is that rheumatoid arthritis is an autoimmune disease. Since lymph nodes represent an essential part of the immune system, rheumatoid arthritis may improve by temporarily "poisoning" the immune system.

Results of studies thus far have been promising—many subjects have noted long-term improvement of their arthritis following treatment. On occasion, this has lasted more than one year. On the other hand, the side effects of radiation therapy are often unpleasant, including, among others, nausea, vomiting, decreased appetite and hair loss. These problems disappear after cessation of therapy. A more serious problem is the development of infections, as the positive effects of the immune system are diminished along with the negative.

Lymph node radiation remains an experimental form of therapy for only the most severe cases of rheumatoid arthritis.

Q: What about copper bracelets?

A: Blood levels of copper in patients with rheumatoid arthritis are higher than normal, so on purely theoretical grounds the bracelet is worthless.

Some people might point to the above observation and suggest eliminating copper from the diet. However, the increased copper level is a result of the inflammatory reaction, not of nutritional aberrations, and cannot be corrected by dietary control.

241

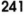

Q: Every year I go to a spa, and my arthritis improves. Is it my imagination? Should I keep going?

A : This question usually comes from my European
patients. In fact, many of them insist on returning
to a spa yearly. They usually come back improved, and
the improvement often lasts for a number of months.

Health spas do more than expose their proponents to
mineral springs. For example, they advocate and provide
a healthy, well-balanced diet. Exercise classes are available and often mandatory. Various types of physical therapy are provided. By definition, the patient is removed
from home and family pressures. So it's not surprising
that most people return from spas feeling refreshed.

Q : I read that bee stings can make arthritis better. Is
it worth it?

A : No, it's not worth it. Rarely, patients with arthritis
who have been stung by bees report a temporary
improvement, no doubt as a result of the production of
various hormones that have an anti-inflammatory effect.

Enterprising individuals have capitalized on this
coincidence and in essence sold bee stings for a profit.
Some who tout this form of therapy claim it takes hundreds, even thousands, of stings to really make a difference. This therapy is potentially dangerous. You may be
allergic to bee venom and not know it; an allergic reaction could have dire consequences.

Q : Someone told me that sex can help arthritis. Is this
true?

A : Believe it or not, it can—but only temporarily. Sex
stimulates the production of various hormones,
such as cortisone and adrenaline. Some of these substances have a natural anti-inflammatory effect and can
reduce pain for a little while. I first became aware of this
after one of my patients returned from a Florida vacation
feeling much better than before she left. When I asked
her to explain her improvement, she said, "The warm
weather, not having to think about my job, and sex." You
can draw your own conclusions—but remember, it's not a
substitute for conventional therapy.

The Nose Knows 28

Scientists are tapping into the mental and emotional powers of scents.

By Carla Kallan

Perhaps it has always been apparent. As plain as the nose on your face. But nobody was paying much attention.

"From an evolutionary point of view, we typically don't think of the nose as very important," says Gary Schwartz, Ph.D., professor of psychology at the University of Arizona. "But it is stuck square in the middle of the face. Why would something that was less relevant to normal activities be so prominent? It implies there is something more important there than we may have realized."

Indeed, scientists are learning that fragrance affects us more than previously thought. New research indicates that smells may influence our minds, our moods and our bodies. But smell remains one of the least understood senses.

Although we know a great deal about the eyes and ears, we only partly understand smell. According to Charles Wysocki, Ph.D., an olfactory scientist at the Monell Chemical Senses Center in Philadelphia, we do know that an odor is first detected by the olfactory epithelium, a sort of receptor sheet located in the nose. This starts a chain of events that leads to an information flow to the olfactory bulb and to the limbic system of the brain, which plays a key role in regulating body functions and the emotions.

Smell, Dr. Wysocki says, is the only sensory system to project directly into the limbic system, making it perhaps our most basic, primitive sense. (Other senses reach the limbic system but travel first to other brain regions.)

Some of the most significant new findings about smell and scent come from William Dember, Ph.D., and Joel Warm, Ph.D., at the University of Cincinnati. They have concluded that scents can keep people more alert and improve performance of routine tasks.

In one study, subjects tackled a 40-minute vigilance

test, which required them to watch a video screen and press a button whenever a certain line pattern appeared. While performing the task, some were intermittently given a whiff of peppermint or muguet (lily of the valley) through oxygen masks. Dr. Dember says that those workers receiving the fragrances performed 25 percent better than those given only whiffs of pure air.

A replication study conducted by Raja Parasuraman, Ph.D., at Catholic University in Washington, D.C., using only peppermint, achieved the same findings. "Maybe what fragrance is doing is raising the level of physiological arousal," Dr. Dember says. Another possibility is that "there's some sort of pharmacologic effect on the centers of the brain that affect alertness, something chemically special." Thus, it is conceivable that certain scents activate specific chemical messengers in the brain, called neurotransmitters.

Although it isn't clear exactly how fragrance works, Dr. Dember believes his study may have practical applications. "Truck drivers, even passenger-car drivers, who need to keep alert while traveling long distances, could find it helpful," he says. An industry group, International Flavors and Fragrances, selected the scents and sponsored this study.

Scents in the Workplace

In Japan, fragrance is already used in the workplace. Shimizu, Japan's largest architectural, engineering and construction firm, has developed an environmental fragrancing system that uses computerized techniques to deliver scents through air-conditioning ducts. The Japanese believe that scents enhance efficiency and reduce stress among office workers.

In one experiment in Japan, 13 key-punch operators were monitored eight hours a day for a month. When the office air was scented with lavender, errors per hour dropped 21 percent. They dropped by 33 percent with a jasmine fragrance, and a stimulating lemon aroma was associated with 54 percent fewer errors.

Junichi Yagi, vice-president of Shimizu's Boston subsidiary, S. Technology Center America, Inc., says the key-punchers enjoyed the fragrances. "They reported feeling better than they did without them," he maintains. Yagi says the fragrances were selected based upon the principles of "aromatherapy," an ancient form of herbal medicine. Aromatherapists believe that essential oils, the distilled essences of flowers, herbs and plants, can be used to make people feel better. Oils such as lavender and chamomile are considered relaxing; lemon and jasmine, stimulating; pine and eucalyptus, invigorating. Scientific evidence to support these claims, however, is still lacking. Aromatherapy is widely practiced in England, France, Belgium, Germany and Switzerland.

Scent Secrets from the Lab

Other research is still in the laboratory phase. Peter Badia, Ph.D., a psychology professor at Bowling Green State University in Ohio, is finding that even when you are sleeping, your nose is wide awake. He's worked with about 100 college subjects in the university sleep lab. Electrodes on test participants monitored brain-wave activity, heart rate, respiration and muscle tension. "What we've determined is that we respond to odors in sleep," Dr. Badia says. "Our tests clearly showed subjects are able to detect odors; typically their heart rate would increase slightly, and their brain waves quicken slightly."

Dr. Badia has discovered that most odors disrupt sleep. Can any fragrance enhance it? Dr. Badia has yet to find one, although he says that heliotropin (a vanilla-and-almond fragrance) is clearly "not disruptive, and might be somewhat beneficial for sleep." Dr. Badia is using scents based upon earlier laboratory research findings and those selected by the Fragrance Foundation, an industry group that sponsored the study.

But Dr. Schwartz thinks that while he was at Yale University he may have found a relaxing scent: spiced apples. Dr. Schwartz conducted the experiments over a five-year period, testing more than 400 subjects.

Dr. Schwartz published findings that he terms "quite remarkable." "We found spiced apple had relaxing effects

245
■

as measured in brain waves, within a minute of [a subject's] smelling the fragrance."

In a separate study, respiration, muscle tension, heart rate and blood pressure were measured as a group of healthy volunteers was asked a series of stressful questions, such as: "The kind of person I find sexually attractive is...?" They received whiffs of spiced apple aroma, while a control group was given bursts of plain air. The spiced apple produced a drop in blood pressure on average of 5 millimeters per person, says Dr. Schwartz.

Dr. Schwartz, now at the University of Arizona, is looking at "subliminal scent"—scent below the level of awareness.

"I think one of the reasons taking trips to pine forests makes us feel so good is the presence of the mixture of molecules in pine," Dr. Schwartz says. "Equally important, if not more important, may be the absence of all these other molecules we're not consciously aware our nose is picking up...smog molecules, gasoline, carpet, paint...which are often putting a great strain on our nervous system."

Dr. Schwartz points to so-called sick buildings as an example. They inhibit the circulation of fresh air, so people instead breathe a veritable soup of man-made chemicals. "The idea is that the nose can detect those molecules and that information is fed to the brain and does activate brain centers to make us feel queasy or uncomfortable," Dr. Schwartz says. "Yet we wouldn't be able to attribute it to any scent we're aware of."

At the Memorial Sloan-Kettering Cancer Center in New York City, William H. Redd, Ph.D., is winding up a study to see if aromas can control stress in people undergoing magnetic resonance imaging (MRI).

"In MRI," Dr. Redd says, "you're put into a...small cylinder...inside a big machine that's a 12×12-foot cube....You have to remain in there as much as an hour and a half, and you're not supposed to move. People have claustrophobic reactions, anxiety and panic attacks."

Dr. Redd says that 10 percent of people react adversely and have to terminate their scans, which means they just wasted about $1,500. "We calculate an average 15-minute delay may result in the loss of $62.5 million in scanning time a year nationwide."

In his study of 85 patients, Dr. Redd found that patients who received the scent of heliotropin during MRI scans experienced 63 percent less anxiety than the control group. The study was presented at the meeting of the Society of Behavioral Medicine in Washington, D.C.

With these and other experiments in progress, it is clear that the study of scent is positively blossoming. "It's definitely on the increase," Dr. Wysocki says. "We've learned a lot, but we're a long way from fully understanding smell. We're still on a great adventure."

Everyday Health Tips

Stop the Sniffles

35 ways to keep your kids feeling good all winter long.

When cold and flu season hits, parents and children need all the TLC they can get. On average, parents have to deal with sniffling, sneezing kids with colds six times a year or more.

And at some point, parents are bound to find themselves taking care of a child with the flu.

And no matter how common the cold is, it's still no fun for any child. Colds arrive slowly, with sneezing, stuffiness, runny nose, thick coughing, raspy throat and sometimes mild fever. Treated or untreated, they last a few days. Flu, on the other hand, comes on like gangbusters.

A child with flu is more likely to have higher fever than he would with a cold, along with headaches, dry cough, chills, sore eyes and muscle pain. We're talking major misery here—lasting about five days. But none of this means that parents are helpless in their attempts to ease the pain and discomfort brought on by sniffle season—their children's and their own.

There are a few tried-and-true remedies that bring relief from the symptoms of colds and flu. (You should also know about a few often-used remedies that don't work.) And you may even be able to reduce the chances of colds and flu striking in the first place.

Here are 35 suggestions to help you survive the siege.

Keeping Viruses at Bay

1. Wash, Wash, Wash ▶ "That's the number-one way to decrease the incidence of colds in day-care situations," says Daniel Shea, M.D., president of the American Academy of Pediatrics. Don't scrub children raw, however. Soap doesn't kill cold or flu viruses but loosens germ-laden oil and deposits on the skin so that running water can carry them away.

Also, little ones tend to put things in their mouth, which is the second most common route of infection. Experts advise under-the-weather parents to scrub up before they handle items such as spoons, teething rings and especially bottles and foods eaten with the fingers.

David Weber, M.D., associate professor of medicine, pediatrics and epidemiology at the University of North Carolina Schools of Medicine and Public Health, adds diapering to the wash-up list. "Make it a habit to wash a child's hands (and your own) after diapering. Children may put their hands under their diapers and then to their faces, spreading infections that way," he says.

2. Teach Children Not to Cover a Sneeze with Their Hands ▶ That actually helps spread colds more than anything else—it simply concentrates the virus in the hand for transfer to another unsuspecting victim, unless your child washes with an antiseptic or antimicrobial soap and water right after sneezing. Tell your child to turn his head away and toward the floor when sneezing. It's also a good idea to teach him to cover his mouth with a disposable tissue while sneezing. Colds are spread best by direct transfer of droplets, or touching contaminated hands, rather than airborne achoos.

3. Break the Sniffling Habit ▶ Children who constantly drip learn to wipe their noses on shirtsleeves and backs of hands, both very convenient spots for passing along germs. Pin packets of tissues to their clothes if need be, or encourage them to ask their teachers for tissues to blow in when they feel their nose running.

4. Show Children How to Blow Their Nose Correctly ▶ They should not pinch both nostrils closed at the same time or blow vigorously. Instead, they should close one nostril and blow through the other gently, or exhale gently through both nostrils. Though it sounds like it's accomplishing something, a loud honk actually may force infectious material deep inside the ears or sinuses, where it can do its dirty work.

5. Dispose of Tissues after Each Use ▶ Don't let germ-laden tissues accumulate in bathrobe pockets or under pillows.

6. Disinfect with Spray or with Wipe Solutions ▶ Go after these high-touch objects: toys, telephones, doorknobs, faucets, toilet handles, countertops. This may do more to help stop the spread of diarrheal diseases than of respiratory diseases, says Dr. Weber. But germs that cause diarrhea can live from minutes to hours on environmental surfaces unless they're carefully wiped away with a disinfectant, he notes.

"If a child drools all over a toy, it will be contagious for a half hour or so, so yes, it's beneficial to wipe it down before another child picks it up," says Donald Goldman, M.D., epidemiologist at the Children's Hospital in Boston.

7. Wash Contaminated Dishes in Hot Water ▶ Then let them air-dry. Add a little sanitizing bleach to the child's laundry.

8. Teach Youngsters Good Hygiene ▶ When youngsters rub their eyes and nose, viruses can enter through any of the passages leading to the respiratory tract—even the tear ducts, which drain into the nasal cavity. "The average person touches his nose, eyes and mouth four to five times an hour," says Dr. Weber. So about every 15 minutes, a cold gets a chance to gain a foothold.

9. Don't Smoke ▶ Don't let your kids be exposed to smoke. It can damage the protective lining of the nose, throat and lungs, making your child more vulnerable to cold and flu germs.

10. Don't Share Toothbrushes! ▶ Be sure each family member has a clearly identifiable toothbrush so you're not sharing viruses.

11. Supply Disposable Cups ▶ Put them in the kitchen and bathroom for use when someone has a cold or the flu. One-use cups help prevent the spread of a virus.

12. If They Feel Well Enough, You Can Send Children Outside to Play, Even in Winter ▶ Cold viruses flourish even in tropical countries, so temperature itself is not a big deal. Colds season is associated with winter months, but that may be because children spend most of the wintertime in hot, dry rooms in close proximity to one another. So the old notion about keeping children out of drafts to prevent colds is simply wrong. However, if they have fever—from either a cold or the flu—you should restrict their activity until at least 24 hours after the fever has subsided.

13. Send Them to School ▶ Even if they're coughing and sneezing, send them—unless they're feverish or feeling really miserable. You don't want them to lose too much school time for a minor illness like a cold.

"If you keep a child home with every cold, that's a significant amount of lost school time," says Dr. Shea. "A child who is well enough to get around the house is well enough to go to school. The severity of the symptoms, not the symptoms themselves, should be your guide." Colds are responsible for 60 million lost days of school each year in the United States.

14. Provide Plenty of Fresh Fruits and Vegetables in a Balanced Diet ▶ While vitamins and minerals can't cure or even prevent a cold directly, they do play an important role in strengthening the body's immune system. Serve whole-grain breads and cereals regularly. Offer low-fat milk and low-fat yogurt. For a free brochure on children's nutrition, send a business-size, self-addressed stamped envelope to: "Growing Up Healthy," Dept. C, American Academy of Pediatrics, P.O. Box 927, Elk Grove Village, IL 60009-0927.

Comforting Strategies

15. Encourage Your Children to Drink Liquids ▶ A little at a time, every five minutes, can get a lot into them. Dehydration can result when kids have fevers, vomiting or diarrhea or when they're stuffed up and have to breathe through their mouths. Offer unchilled fruit juices. Their strong flavors can usually get through to deadened taste buds. Offer these other liquids: weak sweet tea, flat soda pop, liquid fruit-flavored gelatin, plain warm broth. Milk may be hard to keep down, but it doesn't cause mucus, contrary to popular belief.

16. Make Sure Your Little Sufferer Gets Plenty of Rest ▶ Some quiet downtime will help both of you feel better.

17. Feed Your Kids Chicken Soup ▶ It's a plus not only for its nutritious broth but also for its steam, which can cut through mucus.

18. Prop Up Your Child's Head with Pillows ▶ This allows gravity to aid the flow of mucus.

19. Call a Time-Out for Yourself Occasionally ▶ Being a nurse and giver of TLC to an ill child is hard work. Nap when your sick one does. Eat nutritious foods and don't skip meals. If you wear yourself down until you, too, get sick, who's going to take care of you?

Using Medicines Wisely

While there are no cures for the common cold, nonprescription medicines can help lessen the effects of symptoms such as cough, sore throat, fever and congestion.

20. Stick to Children's Remedies ▶ Don't try to downsize doses of adult medicine for a child.

21. Adhere to Dosage Recommendations and Watch That Symptoms Don't Worsen ▶ Be sure to call your doctor when in doubt.

22. Choose a Remedy That Focuses on Just One Symptom ▶ "If the only symptom a child has is a cough, use just a cough suppressant, not a suppressant plus a decongestant," says Dr. Weber. "Medications do

253
∎

have side effects, so you don't want to medicate more than necessary."

23. Know How to Use Cough Medicine Effectively
▶ The best time to use cough medication is when coughing keeps a child awake. The appropriate dose at bedtime can buy your child some much-needed rest, since it may cause drowsiness. But don't medicate productive coughs, which are those that bring up mucus. Since coughing is usually a protective mechanism, there may be hazards from using excessive amounts of cough medicines. If coughing persists, consult your pediatrician.

24. Ignore Antihistamines ▶ They're of no value for children's colds, only for the coldlike symptoms caused by allergies. Colds don't make the body produce histamines.

25. Avoid Camphor and Camphor-Containing Products ▶ Camphor, when ingested, can cause convulsions in children.

26. Avoid Using Menthol- or Eucalyptus-Containing Ointments on Babies and Very Young Children ▶ They are readily absorbed into the bloodstream and can be toxic.

27. Be Careful with Spray Decongestants ▶ If used for more than a few days, they may actually produce a chemical irritation causing the nasal passages to become irritated again.

Dealing with Fever

28. Monitor Your Child's Temperature ▶ Although many parents feel their child's head, the only certain way to ascertain if a child has fever is to take his or her temperature at one of two sites: in the rectum (rectal temperature) or in the mouth (oral temperature). Note: Be sure to use a standard mercury thermometer or a digital thermometer. Fever strips and other methods of measuring temperature can be unreliable. And if you're using a mercury thermometer, don't forget to shake down the thermometer before using it.

29. Use a Rectal Thermometer for Infants and Toddlers ▶ Lay your child over your lap, belly down, and use your forearm to hold the baby still. Spread the buttocks to locate the opening of the rectum. Gently insert the rounded bulb of a special rectal thermometer (the bulb end of a rectal thermometer is thicker and blunter) that's been lubricated with petroleum jelly. It should go about an inch or so into the rectum. Hold the thermometer in place for three minutes. Be sure to use the correct thermometer. Don't use an oral thermometer to take a rectal reading. However, if necessary, a rectal thermometer can be used to take an oral reading. Make sure it is clean (wash with cold water and soap before and after taking reading), and keep it in the mouth longer than usual.

For infants from one to three months old, a temperature of around 99°F is considered normal—99° to 100.5° is a low-grade fever; 100.5° to 101.5° is elevated fever; and 101.5° and above is high fever.

Important: Call a doctor at the first sign of fever in an infant. In a baby under three months of age, a temperature of 100.5° can be significant. But very young babies can be really sick without having fever. That's because an infant's internal thermostat lacks sophistication. When in doubt, call a doctor. When you call the doctor, say which temperature-taking method you used, since different methods yield different temperatures.

For toddlers from 4 to 24 months old, 98.6° is considered normal—100.5° to 101.5° is a low-grade fever; 101.5°+ is elevated fever; and 102°+ is high fever.

30. Use an Oral Thermometer for Toddlers and Older Children ▶ Make sure they are able hold a thermometer in the proper position under their tongue and without biting. For an accurate oral reading, be sure to hold the thermometer in place for three to five minutes.

An oral temperature of 98.6° or less is considered normal—99.5° is a low-grade fever; 100.5° is elevated fever; and 102°+ is high fever.

255
∎

An oral temperature of 102°+ is reason for concern—call a physician. Other reasons to call the doctor: If the fever lasts for more than a couple of days; if the child is vomiting, convulsing or has a headache; if the child just "doesn't look good."

TREAT IT AT HOME— OR PICK UP THE PHONE?

Although viruses—the cause of most of the aches and pains kids have during cold and flu season—resist doctoring, that doesn't mean you shouldn't see your pediatrician or family doctor when illness strikes. Parents should always be on the lookout for the basic symptoms of respiratory trouble: a harsh or persistent cough, a change in breathing (speeding up or becoming more labored), a change in breathing sound (stridor or wheezing), visible retractions or sucking in of the chest when breathing in.

While in some cases there will be nothing serious, these signs and symptoms nevertheless should be taken seriously and reported promptly to a child's doctor.

In general, see the doctor:

When the child's symptoms make him or you uncomfortable. Don't worry about being an alarmist when your child's health is at stake. A "simple" cold or bout of the flu is not always what it seems to be. Even when it is, it can on rare occasions lead to a more serious illness. A sick child is a stressed child, vulnerable to the one-two punch of, say, a cold that leads to an ear infection. The symptoms of some serious, sometimes life-threatening infections may mimic those of a cold or flu. To the untrained eye, nothing dramatic is afoot. Your pediatrician can help you decide if the youngster should be seen immediately in an emergency room or at his or her office.

Treating a Child with Fever

31. Give Your Child Medication ▶ Fevers, unless your child has symptoms indicating that he or she is seriously ill, can be treated at home, usually with chil-

When the child has a fever. "If a child is feverish, it's always wise to see a doctor. He or she can examine the child to distinguish a cold from other upper respiratory conditions or from a secondary bacterial infection," says Georges Peter, M.D., former chairman of the American Academy of Pediatrics' Committee on Infectious Diseases.

Knowing that rheumatic fever is making a comeback sends many parents scurrying to a doctor at the first sniffle. But rheumatic fever is unrelated to colds. It doesn't even masquerade as one. "The manifestations of rheumatic fever that would be most obvious to a parent are fever with joint tenderness or pain," says Dr. Peter.

Rheumatic fever is a complication of a particular strep infection of the throat that can occur in some cases if the preceding strep infection is not adequately treated. It's an inflammatory disease that can strike the heart's valves, causing serious damage.

A throat culture, taken from a feverish child with a sore throat, can differentiate between strep infections and viral causes of these symptoms. If strep is diagnosed, a 10-day course of antibiotics can prevent complications. In most cases, strep infections, even without antibiotics, do not lead to rheumatic fever. While epidemics have occurred in recent years, overall incidence does not appear to have increased.

dren's acetaminophen. (These symptoms include severe headache, lethargy, stiff neck, difficulty breathing, bouts of vomiting or diarrhea and shortness of breath.) Use the recommended dosage or as the pediatrician directs. Treat a high fever (and call the doctor). Treat a lower fever if the child is really uncomfortable. A fever that persists for several days should also be brought to a doctor's attention.

It's a good idea to write down what medications you give your child and when. It's too easy to lose track. Also, keep medications out of the reach of children and make sure all containers have child-safety caps.

32. Avoid Aspirin ▶ Children with flulike illnesses should not be given aspirin because of its association with Reye's syndrome, a serious neurological condition. While some doctors say aspirin has been given a bum rap, noting the extremely rare incidence of Reye's, most say it's better to be safe than sorry. Since what appears to be a cold might actually be flu or chickenpox, it's smarter not to dose anyone under 18 with aspirin. Also, read the label on medications because some children's medications may contain aspirin.

In the rare instance when Reye's does occur, it usually appears as a child recovers from a viral illness. What appears to be a backslide with vomiting, listlessness and changes in personality or behavior may actually be Reye's. If your child was almost back to normal, then shows these symptoms in rapid succession, call your doctor right away.

33. Give the Child a Refreshing Bath ▶ Try this if the fever remains high 30 to 60 minutes after giving acetaminophen. Sponge or bathe the infant or child with tepid water. Cool water should not be used; the temperature contrast could shock his system, since the fever has elevated his body temperature.

Don't sponge the child with alcohol. It can cool the skin too fast, causing shivering, which raises the body temperature again.

While sponging, do not forgo medications. Although

these medications don't act quite as quickly as sponging, their effect lasts longer—usually for a few hours.

34. Don't Overdress ▶ Dress the child in light clothing to prevent heat retention and permit cooling.

35. Be Alert for Seizures Due to High Fever ▶ Called febrile seizures, these terrifying episodes tend to occur with rapidly escalating temperatures in children, especially those from six months to six years old. During a seizure, a child may bend and extend his legs and arms, his eyes may roll back, he may shake all over, and he may not respond to your voice. In some children, a very high fever is needed to provoke a seizure. In others, even a low temperature of 100°F can lead to febrile seizures.

Generally, febrile seizures, although alarming, are not serious if they last less than 15 minutes, or if a series of seizures lasts no more than 15 minutes. Prolonged seizures, however, can cause lasting brain damage. That's why parents should be aware of temperature changes in a sick child. Keeping the child's temperature below the high-fever mark is the best way to prevent seizures.

You can help the child in the midst of one by turning him facedown so saliva won't choke him. Protect and cushion the head, arms and legs. The seizure should be over in three to five minutes. Call the physician if it lasts longer. After the seizure stops, call your pediatrician for advice.

Banish Blisters 30

You can stop the pain of cold and canker sores.

Cold sores (also known as fever blisters) and canker sores sure can be a pain in the mouth.

A canker sore is a small, round, white or yellowish ulcer, or sore, with a red "halo" surrounding it. It forms inside your mouth, usually on your tongue or the inside of your cheek or lip. It lasts only about one to two weeks. But it can make eating or talking uncomfortable and drinking orange juice a hair-raising experience.

A cold sore usually forms outside the mouth—on the lips, and sometimes on the nostrils, fingers or even eyes. (It occasionally can form inside your mouth, most likely on your gums and roof of your mouth.) It's actually a bunch of small ulcers that rupture to form one larger blister. It appears less circular and more red throughout than canker sores. That blister eventually breaks and oozes. A yellow crust forms and finally is shed when the blister heals within seven to ten days, without scarring. Unlike a canker sore, it has a direct known cause—the herpes simplex (almost always type 1) virus.

Now, don't let that "herpes" stuff scare you, says Brad Rodu, D.D.S., associate professor in the school of dentistry at the University of Alabama, Birmingham. "When people hear of herpes, they automatically think of genital herpes (type 2)," he says. "But this is a much different and separate phenomenon."

Though the two viruses are alike in structure, they turn up in different places. The cold-sore virus can be transmitted by shaking hands. The cold-sore virus is so contagious that 20 to 40 percent of Americans are afflicted with cold sores.

Here are some unexpected triggers of cold- and canker-sore attacks.

Cold Sores

Your Grandmother ▶ Or so the story goes. Most of us contracted the cold-sore virus in childhood.

A classic transmission runs as follows: An adult relative who already has the cold-sore virus kisses your baby face. You get the virus, along with a cold sore. Once you've got a cold sore, you can easily spread it. On first contact with the virus, you may get sick with a fever, fatigue and headache.

That all goes away within about two weeks. Then the virus lies dormant in a facial nerve until one of the instigating factors (which we explain below) weakens your body's defenses to it. The result is a cold sore à la Grandma.

Once you already have the virus, a cold sore is only really brought out by one of the other factors below. It's not a new virus you pick up from an infected certain someone.

The Cold, Cruel World ▶ Cold sores can be brought out by fever or illness, hence the names. But the outdoor temperature can play a role, too. Cold wind or hot sunlight can stir up the virus.

When you're going out in the sun, you should always wear sunscreen. But pay special attention to your lips if you're prone to fever blisters. Wear lip sunscreen and a broad-brimmed hat, and sit in the shade of an umbrella.

And skiers, the rush of cold wind while skiing is famous for bringing out blisters. Wear a ski mask.

An Oral Trauma ▶ Your mouth is susceptible to harm from a number of seemingly innocent sources. Hot pizza can burn your mouth, leading to a blister. A rough-edged tooth or a cracked filling can rub the inside of your mouth, eventually causing a sore.

A Dental Visit ▶ Some patients' mouths just seem to have a tendency to develop fever blisters. For them, the trauma that may result from the dentist working in their mouth could weaken their immune system. That can lead to a cold sore. Since you need to go to the dentist, you can't do much to prevent it.

Canker Sores

Irritating Foods ▶ Some people find that their canker sores are related to the foods they eat. Highest on the hit list are cherries, plums, pineapples, tomato products, nuts, chocolate and other sweets.

Try an elimination diet to decide whether your diet is wreaking havoc on your mouth, says Sol Silverman, Jr., D.D.S., professor and chairman of the Division of Oral Medicine at the University of California, San Francisco.

Start by cutting out all salty, acidic or sweet foods. Then reincorporate each at regular intervals. For instance, if your canker sores generally show up every four weeks, wait a month before adding the first item back into your diet. If that doesn't give you a problem, move on to the next item the following month. Notice when the sores develop. You might be able to locate a canker-causing ingredient in your diet.

Your Nervous Habit ▶ If you bite the inside of your cheek, you may be encouraging sores to form. Try chewing sugarless gum instead of your cheek.

Stress ▶ Canker sores may proliferate when you're under psychological stress. The standard example is students around exam time being more prone to developing canker sores.

Certain Diseases ▶ People can get sores from a variety of diseases that affect the mouth, says Dr. Rodu. Two are Crohn's disease (a gastrointestinal disorder) and Behçet's syndrome, an autoimmune disease that affects the skin, mouth and eyes.

Keep an eye on sores in or around the mouth that can't be identified and don't heal quickly. There's always the chance that lingering blisters or ulcers are precancerous lesions. See a dentist or physician if a sore lasts more than a few weeks.

Living with Canker and Cold Sores

Experts say there's no real cure for either a cold or canker sore once it's in the works. But you can treat each attack to ease discomfort and even improve appearance.

If used early on, some over-the-counter medications can be effective in keeping the size of the cold sore small. And keeping a cold sore moist with petroleum jelly or ointment can help prevent cracking (which would make it look and feel worse) after the blister breaks. Avoid squeezing or picking it—it can become infected. (If a cold

sore does get infected, see your dent[...]
with a prescription antibiotic ointmen[...]

For canker sores, your dentist can [...]
corticosteroid, which will reduce inflan[...]
ness and induce healing. He can also g[...]
medication to coat the canker sore and[...]
irritation for several hours. There are also[...]
counter gels and rinses that ease pain.

Meanwhile, avoid spicy or acidic foods[...] an
antacid product, such as an antacid tablet (which can
neutralize mouth acids that irritate the sores). And avoid
antiseptic mouthwashes or antiseptic throat lozenges,
because they could irritate the area.

Whatever you do, don't try to ease your pain by
putting aspirin on a canker sore, says Dr. Rodu. Aspirin
is extremely acidic and can cause another, even bigger
ulcer in the mouth.

Pulling the Plug   31

Simple tips for keeping
your ears free of waxy buildups.

At first, Jennifer Blythe thought her four-year-old
son Nathan was just not listening to her. She'd call him
to come inside, and he'd keep right on playing, as if he
were "Mommy deaf." But when she scolded him, his look
of bewilderment made her concerned. "It was obvious he
really didn't hear me," she says. "I thought it might be
caused by a hearing problem."

Her pediatrician made a quick and comforting diagnosis. "It was earwax," says Jennifer, a mother of two in
suburban Philadelphia. "Nathan had tons of it! It seems
to run in the family. My husband, Shawn, had so many
hearing problems when he was in college that he went to
the school nurse. He said she worked on his ear for a long
time before she finally dislodged a ball of wax. He said he
could hear so well after that, it was actually painful."

Cleaning and
Protecting the Ear

Earwax doesn't get talked about much—and with good reason. As conversation fodder, it falls somewhere between dandruff and foot odor. But it is the result, after all, of a natural bodily process. Earwax, or cerumen, as it is known medically, is a natural and necessary secretion meant to clean and protect the ear. As such, most of the time doctors recommend that you just leave it alone.

But as with all natural processes, this one can go awry. Too much cerumen can collect in an ear canal, clogging it and leading to a problem with temporary hearing loss. Children with impacted earwax may begin having trouble in school.

Older people may become depressed if they regard the hearing loss as a sign they're succumbing to old age and decay. Suddenly, a problem that sounds like the punch line to a joke can take a serious turn.

Doctors don't know what causes excess earwax accumulation, which tends to be a recurrent problem. But they do know there are certain factors involved that may cause the cerumen to collect.

Factors That Make
Things Worse

First, and most common, is the use of cotton swabs, bobby pins, matchsticks, fingernails or anything small enough to penetrate the ear canal. People tend to use these items to try to remove earwax, thinking that they're helping to prevent the problem from getting worse.

Actually they're exacerbating it. Instead of removing earwax, they're pushing it in. Which is why doctors agree with grandmothers and insist that "you never should put anything smaller than an elbow in your ear."

Earwax—just enough of it—is good for you. Formed in the glands of the outer part of the ear canal, it traps sand, dust and insects (like gnats and ticks) and keeps these tiny intruders away from the sensitive eardrum. It repels water and serves as an antibacterial agent, helping to ward off infections of the ear canal. It also moisturizes the skin of the outer ear and ear canal, preventing dryness and itching.

The cells of the ear grow and migrate outward from the eardrum to the external part of the ear. As they move along the ear canal, sort of like a moving walkway, they transport earwax and any foreign bodies the wax may have snared. Normally this dried or accumulated earwax winds up outside the ear canal, where it dries and falls out, or it can be wiped away easily by a finger wrapped round a washcloth or tissue—the only safe and approved way of removing normal earwax.

But taking long showers in the name of cleanliness isn't going to help. If you have an earwax problem, water isn't your friend. Swimming, long showers or any other activity that might introduce water into the ear canal could also cause earwax impaction, especially among people who are prone to this problem. Water can make the earwax swell into a plug.

David N. F. Fairbanks, M.D., an otolaryngologist and spokesperson for the American Academy of Otolaryngology–Head and Neck Surgery, suggests that his patients who have a history of earwax impaction come to see him to get their ears cleaned out at least once a year, in late May—right before the start of the swimming season.

Another doctor tells the story of a 16-year-old who complained of hearing loss in his left ear. After taking a brief history of the patient, the doctor learned that the young man customarily took 30-minute showers, so he wasn't surprised to see a swollen earwax plug when he looked into the teenager's ear canal.

The kind of earwax your glands produce may also contribute to the problem. In young people, particularly children, earwax is usually soft—wet, sticky and honey-colored. As people get older, their cerumen sometimes gets harder. This flaky, dry, dandrufflike earwax does not move along the ear canal as easily as the softer kind. It may also be more susceptible to swelling when it comes in contact with water.

265

Some people may produce an overabundance of earwax, while others may have particularly small ear canals. And those individuals who wear hearing aids may find that device to be part of their wax problem, because it can prevent the easy flow of earwax out of the ear.

Fixing the Problem

Whatever the cause, impacted earwax should be removed. This can often be accomplished at home, but not until you're diagnosed as having an earwax problem.

Once you know you have a tendency toward earwax buildup, there are certain steps you can take to clear it up and prevent future accumulation. But before you embark on any of these steps, make sure your eardrum is intact and you have no history of ear infections, ear surgery or eardrum perforation (puncture).

First, if your ear feels full and your hearing hindered, you might try putting some eardrops in your ear to soften the wax. This earwax solvent could be mineral oil, baby oil or over-the-counter or prescription eardrops. Most doctors don't seem to prefer one product over another, but some experts suggest that oil-based drops are more effective than water-based drops for softening the wax in preparation for ear washing. Water-based drops are more likely to produce infection. For adults, put six to eight drops in the ear twice a day for a few days. For infants or children, consult a physician first.

The drops may be enough to relieve the symptoms. But be prepared for potential side effects. "When we gave Nathan the drops, he woke up the next morning screaming," Jennifer recalls. "He wasn't in pain. It's just that they worked so well there was earwax all over his pillow. It scared him." If you are prone to earwax buildup, you might want to use eardrops on a weekly basis to keep cerumen from accumulating.

If the eardrops alone don't do the trick, you can irrigate the ear to flush out the remaining wax. To do this you need a rubber syringe and a basin of warm water (the warmer, the better, as earwax melts at body temperature). Although you can irrigate your ear by yourself, you might want to ask someone to help you out, since a third hand would be useful.

After applying the eardrops, fill the syringe with warm water. Then follow these steps in order.

1. Pull your earlobe up and back to straighten out the ear canal.

2. Place the tip of the syringe no closer than 1/2 inch from the hole in your ear, and squirt some water into the ear canal.

3. Tilt your head to the side to let the water drain from your ear. Be sure to remove as much water as possible by turning your ear down and pulling and wiggling it.

4. Finally, place an eardropper full of rubbing alcohol into the irrigated ear. The alcohol absorbs all remaining water and sterilizes the ear to prevent infection.

Since wax plugs are often tightly packed in the ear canal, you may have to repeat this procedure 10, 20, 50, even 100 times ("which is why my patients come to me to have this done," says Dr. Fairbanks). After a while, you should notice that the water coming back out of your ear has darkened as the melted earwax begins to flow out.

If this procedure seems too arduous to handle on your own, you can always go to your physician, who will irrigate the ear, use a suction tube to vacuum it out or use a tiny instrument to pull out the plug. Once the wax is gone, your hearing should improve dramatically.

The
Good
Life

Put Insomnia to Bed 32

A step-by-step plan for getting a good night's sleep every night.

By Gregg D. Jacobs, Ph.D.

Editor's Note: Sleep is something we take for granted— until it plays hard to get. Then we're willing to do just about anything for a few winks. At the Mind/Body Medical Institute in Boston, however, treatment for chronic sleeplessness begins by weaning sufferers off addictive sleeping pills. Under the direction of Harvard professor and relaxation expert Herbert Benson, M.D., the institute offers instruction in a total self-care program involving behavior modification and training in the relaxation response. Eighty percent of those who've been through the program report sleep success. Now you, too, can learn the techniques.

Most individuals suffer occasional sleepless nights or periods of poor sleep during stressful life events, such as job or home difficulties, pregnancy, a wedding, an illness or a death. For some, occasional sleeping problems can evolve into chronic insomnia. Over 100 million Americans are estimated to have occasional sleep problems, and about 1 in 6 has chronic insomnia and considers it a serious problem.

Fortunately, a significant amount of research devoted to sleep and insomnia over the past 25 years has uncovered many things you can do to improve your sleep. In fact, because of side effects from sleep medications, behavioral techniques are now considered the most effective form of treatment for chronic insomnia.

Our program incorporates a number of clinically proven behavioral techniques for managing insomnia. Our research suggests that this program results in significant improvements in sleep in about 80 percent of our patients. To obtain the benefits, however, it is necessary to practice these techniques in the sequential, stepwise manner in which they are presented.

Each set of techniques requires about one to two weeks of practice before it begins to regularly affect your sleep. Once you are practicing one set of techniques consistently, begin to practice the next set.

Overcoming insomnia cannot be done quickly. Too many people abandon a behavioral technique after two or three nights if it doesn't produce any immediate change in their sleep. Our behavioral self-help program requires time, patience and persistence. Furthermore, although the changes resulting from behavioral interventions may be slower than those produced by medication, they are more enduring and effective.

If you are persistent and use these techniques regularly over a ten-week period, you should significantly improve your sleep.

What Is Insomnia?

There is no standard definition of insomnia, since the amount of sleep required for feeling rested varies widely among individuals. Some feel rested with four hours of sleep, while others require ten. According to Dr. Patricia Lacks of Washington University in St. Louis, an arbitrary definition of insomnia may include any of the following.

Sleep-Onset Insomnia ▶ Difficulty falling asleep defined by an average of at least 30 minutes to fall asleep.

Sleep-Maintenance Insomnia ▶ Difficulty staying asleep as defined by an average awake time after falling asleep totaling more than 30 minutes per night, or early-morning awakening before the desired wake-up time with an inability to fall back asleep.

Poor Quality of Sleep ▶ Insomnia can be caused by stress or other behavioral factors, such as unrealistic sleep expectations, inappropriate scheduling of sleep, trying too hard to sleep, consuming caffeine, inadequate exercise and a number of other behavioral factors. Insomnia can also be caused by depression, a medical problem or alcohol or drug use. Before beginning this self-help program, get a complete physical history and medical examination from your physician. The techniques discussed here are not appropriate for insomnia caused by depression, alcohol or drug use or a medical condition.

Take a moment to reflect on your sleep pattern.

■ Do you have difficulty staying asleep?

■ Do you feel your sleep is of poor quality?

■ Do you have a combination of these types of sleep patterns? If yes, reflect on behaviors that may influence your sleep pattern.

■ Do you worry or feel anxious at bedtime?

■ Do you try too hard to sleep?

■ Do you smoke or consume caffeine near bedtime?

■ Do you spend too much time in bed?

■ Do you get too little exercise?

■ Do you have an inconsistent sleep schedule?

The Effects of Sleep Loss

The effects of sleep loss are subject to a number of popular misconceptions. The belief that everyone must sleep eight hours a night is a myth.

According to Dr. Peter Hauri at the Mayo Clinic in Rochester, Minnesota, adults average about 7 to 7½ hours of sleep per night, and many individuals function effectively with 4 to 6 hours of sleep. In fact, 20 percent of the population (slightly more in men) sleep less than 6 hours per night. Another significant fact is that sleep time decreases with age.

Contrary to popular belief, the human nervous system has a remarkable tolerance for sleep loss, at least on a temporary basis. As Dr. Hauri notes, one night of total sleep deprivation makes healthy young volunteers sleepy but has remarkably little effect on their day's performance.

Dr. Claudio Stampi, an expert on sleep research, observes that most individuals can maintain their usual performance with 60 to 70 percent of their normal sleep. If you are an 8-hour sleeper, this means your performance at work will not suffer significantly if you get 4½ to 5½ hours of sleep.

In fact, a study conducted by Dr. Jeffrey Sugerman, Dr. John Stern and Dr. James Walsh on sleep and insomnia found that individuals suffering from insomnia perform as well on tests of mental performance as good sleepers.

For moderate sleep loss, then, the perception is as important as the amount lost. So don't be afraid of insomnia. The less you fear insomnia, and the less you appraise sleep loss as stressful, the better you will sleep, and the better you will feel the next day.

Now that you understand some basic facts about sleep and insomnia, let us turn to the first set of behavioral techniques to improve your sleep.

Take a moment to assess your reaction to sleep loss.
■ Are you overly concerned about getting eight hours of sleep?

■ Do you panic about sleep loss?

■ Do you get angry and frustrated when you cannot sleep?

■ Do you tell yourself you will be unable to function the next day?

Improving Daytime and Before-Sleep Behaviors

Practice these steps daily.

Step 1 ▶ Under the supervision of a physician, gradually eliminate the use of sleeping pills. The effects achieved by most sleep medications are only temporary, since they lose their effectiveness after two to four weeks of continued use. They also decrease deep sleep and dream sleep, so that while you may fall asleep faster, your sleep will be of poorer quality. Besides disrupting sleep, sleep medications are usually not eliminated from the body by morning and produce a "hangover" effect, which can decrease daytime alertness and impair thinking. People also tend to develop tolerance for the medication and need increasingly larger doses. Additionally, psychological or physical dependence can develop if the medication is used for an extended period. Finally, when you stop using them, many sleep medications result in a temporary rebound insomnia that can be worse than the initial insomnia! So, if you must take a sleeping pill, limit yourself to one per week.

Step 2 ▶ Reduce your consumption of alcohol and caffeine. Alcohol disrupts sleep by reducing deep sleep and dream sleep; it should not be consumed within two hours of bedtime. Caffeine is a powerful stimulant and should not be consumed within six hours of bedtime. Many foods, beverages and medications contain caffeine—read the product labels carefully. If you smoke, stop. Nicotine is a stimulant, and nonsmokers fall asleep more quickly than smokers.

Step 3 ▶ Establish a regular aerobic exercise program. As suggested by Dr. Hauri, people who have difficulty sleeping tend to lead more sedentary lives than good sleepers, and we now know that physical inactivity may contribute to insomnia (by inhibiting our normal and rhythmic increases and decreases of body temperature).

Regular exercise in the late afternoon or early evening eliminates this problem because it makes your body temperature rise and then fall (as you cool down). Dr. Deborah Sewitch at the Griffin Hospital in Derby, Connecticut, observes that this aids your sleep because decreasing body temperature facilitates the onset of sleep and promotes deep sleep. However, exercise early in the morning does not affect sleep, and exercise within three hours of bedtime may stimulate you, which can make it more difficult to fall asleep.

For many individuals, brisk walking in the late afternoon or early evening is sufficient to increase core body

273

temperature. You should exercise at least three to four times per week in order to affect your sleep consistently.

Step 4 ▶ Plan tomorrow's activities, complete phone calls and personal business, and review the day's events early in the evening so that two hours prior to bedtime can serve as a relaxing, wind-down period. Activities during this transition between waking and sleeping might include reading or watching television. A light carbohydrate snack during your wind-down period may help you sleep, because carbohydrates increase the production of serotonin, the brain chemical responsible for sleep.

Step 5 ▶ Make sure your sleeping environment is conducive to sleep. Minimal levels of light and sound aid sleep. For many individuals, the hum of a fan or an air conditioner or a commercially available sound conditioner aids sleep. Also, make sure the temperature of your bedroom is comfortable. In general, a cooler room temperature facilitates sleep, since this helps decrease your core body temperature.

Step 6 ▶ Reduce your intake of fluids after 8:00 P.M. to help reduce any chance you might have of waking up at night because of a full bladder.

Practice these techniques regularly until they become an integral part of your daily and before-sleep routine. This will probably require at least two weeks of daily practice.

Take a moment to list sleep-hygiene behaviors that might interfere with your sleep pattern. Then list steps you might find useful to improve your sleep-hygiene behaviors.

Scheduling Your Sleep

One of the most important ways to improve your sleep is to reduce your time in bed. It is common for poor sleepers to extend time in bed, especially after a poor night of sleep, in order to "catch up on sleep." However, as Dr. Hauri notes, the more time you spend in bed, the more difficulty you will have falling asleep, and the lighter and poorer your sleep will be. By reducing that time, you will be drowsier at bedtime, you can consolidate and deepen your sleep, and you can create a slight sleep debt that makes it easier to fall asleep and sleep more deeply the next night.

Step 1 ▶ Reduce your time in bed to no more than six to seven hours. For most people, this means delaying bedtime by about one hour. If you become drowsy earlier in the evening, use activity to ward off drowsiness—move around your house, socialize, do some light cleaning—anything to keep you slightly active. Spending too much time in bed is the most common mistake a person with insomnia can make. Cutting down that time is crucial to improving your sleep.

Step 2 ▶ Get up at about the same time every day (including weekends), even if you have had a poor night's sleep. This helps maintain a consistent circadian rhythm—the 24-hour internal body rhythm or cycle—that keeps humans awake during the day and asleep (usually) at night. With time, the hour that you become drowsy will become more consistent. As noted by Dr. Charles Reynolds at the University of Pittsburgh School of Medicine, getting up at the same time each day and not sleeping in also promotes a slight sleep debt that will make it easier to fall asleep and sleep more deeply.

Step 3 ▶ Use prior wakefulness to regulate when you get drowsy and how deeply you sleep. The longer you are awake (that is, the earlier you get up), the quicker you fall asleep, and the deeper you sleep, that night. If you have an important meeting early Monday morning and want the best chance of getting to sleep at a reasonable time Sunday night, get up earlier Sunday morning.

Step 4 ▶ Do not nap longer than one hour, especially late in the day, since naps of this length can make you less sleepy at bedtime. Naps under 60 minutes, however, may be beneficial after a sleep-deprived night, especially around 3:30 in the afternoon. According to Dr. Scott Campbell and Dr. Juergen Zulley at the Max Planck Institute in Munich, Germany, our mood and performance decline in mid-afternoon due to a biological need for sleep. A short nap can satisfy the need and usually will not affect sleep onset.

Allow yourself at least two weeks to integrate sleep-scheduling techniques into your daily routine. At the end of this period, you should be practicing both sleep-hygiene and sleep-scheduling techniques regularly.

Take a moment to reflect on your sleep schedule.

■ What time do you usually go to bed?

■ What time do you usually get up?

■ How much time do you spend in bed?

■ Do you nap frequently?

■ Identify several strategies to improve your sleep scheduling.

Stimulus-Control Training

For most people, the bed and bedroom are associated with relaxation, drowsiness and sleep. For many poor sleepers, however, the bed and bedroom have become conditioned cues for mental arousal, sleeplessness and frustration because they are used for many activities other than sleep, including reading work-related materials, talking on the phone, worrying and, most important, trying too hard to sleep. Interestingly, some individuals with insomnia sleep well everywhere except their own bedroom, including other rooms in their house, in front of the television or even in a sleep laboratory!

The goal of stimulus-control training is to teach you to reassociate the bed and bedroom with relaxation, drowsiness and sleep. Most important, stimulus control can teach you not to try to sleep, which is one of the biggest mistakes anyone who has difficulty sleeping can make.

Based on our research and clinical work with people who sleep poorly, we have developed a modified version of the stimulus-control technique originally developed by Dr. Richard Bootzin at Northwestern University in Evanston, Illinois.

Step 1 ▶ Use your bedroom only for pleasurable, relaxing activities and sleep. Do not use your bedroom for any stressful activities. Furthermore, do not use your bed in the evening until bedtime. The goal is to associate your bedroom and bed with relaxation and sleep only.

Step 2 ▶ Go to bed only when drowsy, even if that moment comes later than your new delayed bedtime. The goal is to associate bedtime and your bed with drowsiness.

Step 3 ▶ When you are quite drowsy, get into bed and relax for 15 to 20 minutes by reading, listening to music or watching television until you are very drowsy. Then turn out the lights with the intention of going to sleep. If you are not asleep within 20 to 25 minutes, do not try to sleep! The harder you try, the more you will stay awake. Instead, open your eyes and read—a book reading light works well—or watch TV until you are drowsy again, then turn out the lights to sleep again. Repeat this procedure as often as necessary. If you regularly repeat this process three or four times, you are going to bed too early.

If you are wide awake and your mind is very active, you are probably better off getting out of bed and leaving your bedroom. This is especially appropriate if you sleep well everywhere (including other rooms in your own home) except your bedroom, or if you tend to try to go back to sleep too soon when you stay in bed. Engage in quiet, relaxing activity until you begin to feel drowsy again, then return to your bedroom with the intention of going to sleep. Repeat this procedure as often as necessary until you fall asleep.

Take a moment to reflect on any of your bedtime behaviors that are conditioned cues for wakefulness, mental arousal and frustrations that interfere with your ability to sleep.

277

- Do you use the bedroom for nonrelaxing activities?

- Do you go to bed when you are not really drowsy?

- Do you continue to try to sleep if you are still awake after 25 minutes?

After identifying these behaviors, identify strategies to help you reassociate the bed and bedtime with relaxation, drowsiness and sleep.

Stimulus control is one of the most effective behavioral techniques for improving sleep but also one of the most difficult to master. Many people want to go to bed before they are drowsy, and many have difficulty with not trying to sleep. At least two weeks are often needed to begin mastering stimulus-control techniques. Without consistent usage for at least two weeks, you will not learn to associate your bed and bedroom with relaxation, drowsiness and sleep. Practice stimulus-control techniques every night!

Techniques to Elicit the Relaxation Response

Practicing the relaxation response during the day can reduce the daytime physical and mental arousal that may disrupt sleep. In addition, research by Dr. Kenneth Lichstein and Dr. Thomas Rosenthal suggests that bedtime mental arousal—worrying, planning tomorrow's activities or anxiety about falling asleep—can significantly disrupt sleep.

Our research suggests that the relaxation response reduces mental arousal by producing slower brain-wave activity. Normally, you do not fall asleep when eliciting the relaxation response because you are sitting up. However, practicing the relaxation-response instructions at bedtime while lying down can help you fall asleep.

Do not attempt to use the relaxation response to fall asleep until you feel comfortable with these techniques, because trying too hard to relax may actually disrupt sleep. To prevent this from occurring, do not practice the relaxation response at bedtime until you have practiced it during the day for at least two weeks. Then try it at bedtime, after turning off the lights and closing your eyes. If you have little mental arousal at bedtime, you may not need the relaxation response at this time. However, our experience suggests that most individuals with insomnia benefit from this approach.

When you begin to practice the relaxation response at bedtime, combine it with stimulus control. That is, go to bed only when drowsy, distract yourself for 15 to 20 minutes, then use the relaxation-response instructions after you lie down, turn off the lights and close your eyes. You may find you are drowsy enough to fall asleep before completing the relaxation-response instructions.

However, if you are still awake after 25 minutes, do not continue to use the relaxation-response instructions; open your eyes and read or distract yourself until drowsy again. Then close your eyes and use the relaxation-response instructions again. Repeat this process until you fall asleep. If your mind is very active, you may be better off getting out of bed and going to another room until you are drowsy.

If you awaken in the middle of the night, elicit the relaxation response to help you fall back to sleep. However, if you do not fall back to sleep within 25 minutes, open your eyes and read or distract yourself until drowsy. Leave the room only if you are wide awake and your mind is very active. The key to successful relaxation-response practice at bedtime is to not try too hard. The relaxation response requires a passive approach of letting relaxation happen. As you develop this skill, your ability to reduce mental arousal at bedtime will improve.

Maintaining Improvement

If you give yourself a few weeks to master each set of self-help techniques and practice them regularly, your sleep should improve significantly. Be tolerant of occasional sleepless nights, however, and remember that even good sleepers have nights of poor sleep. If your sleep does not improve, getting an evaluation from a sleep clinic at one of your local hospitals would probably be a good idea.

Finally, be sure to continue practicing your self-help techniques so that they become a permanent part of your daily behaviors. Follow-up data from a number of research studies suggest that people who use these behavioral techniques regularly rarely relapse into old sleeping patterns. In fact, one-year follow-ups show that improvement stays the same or increases for people who continue their sleep-healthy habits. Regular practice is worth the effort. Not only will your sleep improve, but your sense of control over sleep will improve as well.

LEARN TO RELAX FOR BETTER SLEEP

To elicit the physiological state called the relaxation response, you need to practice a technique that helps you "let go" more deeply than most of us can without such help. The basic steps are as follows.

Step 1: Pick a focus word or short phrase that is firmly rooted in your personal belief system. For example, a Christian might choose the opening of Psalm 23, *The Lord is my shepherd*; a Jew, *Shalom*; a Muslim, *Allah*; a nonreligious person, a neutral word or phrase like *one* or *peace* or *love*.

Step 2: Sit quietly in a comfortable position.

Step 3: Close your eyes.

Step 4: Relax your muscles.

Step 5: Breathe slowly and naturally, and as you do, repeat your focus word or phrase as you exhale.

Step 6: Assume a passive attitude. Do not worry about how well you're doing. When other thoughts come to mind, simply say to yourself, "Oh, well," and gently return to the repetition.

Step 7: Continue for 10 to 20 minutes.

Step 8: Practice the technique a minimum of once or twice daily.

Mastering the Senior Years

You can supercharge your retirement with new friends, new places and new challenges.

Retirement is generally viewed as a time of intellectual rustiness, life relegated to the mental slow lane. But your retired years don't have to be that way.

You can have the same intellectual sharpness and zest for living at 75 that you have at 55, if you put your mind to it—and start today. Here's how the experts say people in their preretirement years can prep their mental machinery for years and years of rust-free action.

Embrace Mental Challenges

"The adage 'use it or lose it' applies to the mind as well as the muscles," says Marian Diamond, Ph.D., professor of neurosciences at the University of California, Berkeley. Just as muscles grow with physical exercise, the nerve cells in the brain expand with mental challenges.

Nerve cells have branches called dendrites that act like miniature telephone lines, allowing the cells to communicate with each other. Research shows that the brain cells of animals housed in intellectually enriched environments—with stimulating toys and the company of other animals—have more of these dendrites than the brain cells of animals kept in toyless solitude.

"The same goes for humans," says Dr. Diamond. "Studies show that the area in the brain devoted to word understanding is significantly larger in the average college graduate than in the average high-school graduate. Why? Because college graduates spend more time working with words."

Dr. Diamond urges people in their midcareer years to challenge themselves intellectually every day with anything from crossword puzzles to learning new languages to taking new jobs. "Recently, at age 64," she says, "I took a new job. I became the director of the Lawrence Hall of Science at Berkeley, which designs science and math curricula for the nation's elementary schools. I wanted the stimulation and challenge, and I couldn't think of a better way to keep my mind from getting rusty than to devote myself to getting children interested in and excited about math and science."

Just be careful not to overdo the mental stimulation. When the toys used to enrich experimental animal environments are changed too often, the animals' brains do not develop as much as those with less stimulation, Dr. Diamond says. "Too much stimulation loses its value. By all means, enrich your mental life, but allow yourself adequate time to assimilate new information."

Harness the Mental Power of Exercise

While your brain needs mental stimulation to stay sharp, a growing body of evidence shows that it needs one other thing as well: exercise.

According to a study conducted by Robert Dustman, Ph.D., a Salt Lake City research psychologist at the VA Medical Center, a little aerobic exercise can improve short-term memory, creativity and reaction time.

And that's not all. Other research points to the strong possibility that regular workouts may sharpen your sense of taste, stave off depression and enhance your reasoning abilities. The best part of these studies is that they weren't conducted on a bunch of cleat-footed youngsters. The razor-sharp folks that were tested here ranged from 55 to 91.

Take Time to Encourage Your Interests

Difficult as this may seem, carve out some time—even a few hours a week—when you can step back from your daily responsibilities and indulge in some non-work activity you truly enjoy. This doesn't mean heading for the hammock with a back scratcher and a beer. It means getting involved with a hobby—especially one that has the potential of becoming more than just a hobby.

"Hobbies are enriching at any age," says 65-year-old Ron Lawrence, M.D., neurologist at the UCLA School of Medicine. "But they become crucial as retirement looms because they enhance self-esteem and confer a sense of identity at a time when your work identity may be disappearing."

Dr. Lawrence enjoys several hobbies: photography, painting, astronomy and ham radio. He says the best time to get serious about hobbies is during the midcareer years when you generally feel sure of your interests and usually have some money to indulge them somewhat.

In addition to enjoyment, hobbies present brain-preserving mental challenges and opportunities to make new friends. And the sense of accomplishment that comes from mastering anything from baking to woodworking helps offset the loss of career accomplishments during retirement.

"Hobbies and social involvement are especially important to Type A men," says psychologist Allen Elkin, Ph.D., director of the Stress Management and Counseling Center in New York City.

"A client of mine retired a very rich man at the age of 50, but quickly became depressed because he had lost his job identity. Type A's can't simply lie on a beach. Anyone who derives most of their identity from their profession is going to need other sources of self-esteem to fall back on when they leave that profession behind."

Make Time for Each Other

"The average midcareer couple spends only about ten minutes a day talking to each other," Dr. Elkin says. "Retirement greatly expands that time, and problems can develop if spouses don't have activities that they can enjoy together."

The trick is to start exploring joint activities now.

283

That way you'll not only find out what tickles your co-fancy, but also you'll pick up just enough expertise to become truly excited at the prospect of the extra time retirement will provide to hone your skills.

Maybe it's skiing. Golf. Ballroom dancing. Even building a house. The possibilities are limitless.

But one thing is for sure: Mutual interests help keep you mutually interested in each other.

Cherish Old Friends

You might be the most mentally alive, intellectually supercharged person on earth, but that can be cold comfort if you feel alone, isolated and depressed.

When was the last time you contacted your old high-school best friend? College roommate? Favorite cousin? Army buddy? Or that valued co-worker who moved away?

"Some letting go is inevitable and healthy," says Dr. Elkin. "But old friends provide valuable emotional grounding. Their perspectives on your past can help you solve problems in the present and plan for the future. And their evolving interests can introduce you to stimulating new activities and new people you might enjoy."

Keeping in touch also gives you more people and places to visit—now and after you retire.

Make New Friends

As the years pass, it often seems harder and harder to make new friends. Part of the problem is that people tend to feel constrained by family and career responsibilities. They have much less time to "hang out" like they used to. But equally important, after 55, people often fall into emotional ruts and stop reaching out to others who they might find intellectually stimulating.

"One of the great things about hobbies, classes and organizations is that they introduce you to new people who share your interests," Dr. Elkin says. "Those new friends not only make your shared activity more enjoy-able, they also expand your personal network. You can meet their friends, and some of them might become your friends as well."

Close ties to family and friends do a great deal more than make your life—both now and after retirement—more fulfilling. Social support just might extend your life. In a classic experiment, researchers at the University of California, Berkeley, asked several thousand residents of Alameda County, California, to complete an extensive lifestyle questionnaire. After about ten years, they compared the answers of those who'd died with those still alive. Social connectedness correlated strongly with survival.

Those who'd died tended to be considerably more socially isolated than those who'd survived.

Use Vacations as Retirement Test-Runs

You've got money to spend, time to kill and the chance to spend more than 10 or 15 uninterrupted minutes with your spouse.

The fact that vacation and retirement bear such a resemblance can be turned to your advantage. Why not use your next few vacations to scout out new terrain and find your potential retirement paradise?

"I love to travel," says retirement specialist L. Malcolm Rodman, "but I noticed that after a certain point in my life I stopped viewing destinations as just exotic places to visit and started to seriously consider them as possible places to live when I retire." Of course, if you're going to do a bit of scouting, you may want to keep a few of Rodman's guidelines in mind.

■ If the area is a tourist attraction, visit it in the off-season. "Try Florida in the summer or Maine in the winter and see if you still like the area when it's unpopular with the rest of the world," says Rodman.

■ Ask local residents what they think are the most problematic challenges of the locale. You may find that the Arizona heat isn't half as bad as the sandstorms that'll rip your skin.

■ Make a recreational checklist and see if the area meets your needs. Green Mountain Falls, Colorado, may be wonderful for hiking, but the closest thing you'll find to a symphony orchestra may be the Hooterville Jug Band.

■ Look for like-minded people. Does the community have a house of worship that's your brand? Are you a sensitive, artistic sort about to move to an area where woodchuck juggling is considered high art?

If you have nothing in common with the people around you, the risk of isolation is high.

■ Does the community offer adequate medical services? Most places do these days. But if you're dreaming of a cabin in the northwestern corner of Montana, you may want to consider just how far away help may be in case of an emergency.

A change of locale alone won't necessarily rustproof your retirement. But add in a pinch of mental stimulation, a dash of exercise, a teaspoon of camaraderie and a whole lot of fun with a spouse, and you'll have just the kind of polish you need to keep your mind, and your outlook, shiny and new for many years to come.

Index

295

∎

297

■